Painful Sex No More!

A Practical Guide to Pain-Free Intercourse and Path to Sexual Wellness

PELVICPROTHERAPY

Sandi Smith, PT

Global Book Publishing

Painful Sex No More!
Sandi Smith

ISBN: 978-1-956193-73-2
Book Design & Publishing done by:
Global Book Publishing
www.globalbookpublishing.com

Medical Disclaimer: Although this book is intended to be a guide book to lead you down to the path to pain free intercourse, it is not intended to diagnose, treat or counsel in any way. I am not a medical doctor, psychologist or sexologist. In the pages that follow there are times that I recommend seeking professionals, such as MD's or licensed mental health counselors. As a licensed physical therapist I follow the practice act of my state of Florida that is set in place by the Florida State Board of Physical Therapy to protect the public.

You will also find some personal stories that are included to help you understand the magnitude of how many women have this condition. The stories are based on the truth about real patients just like you. Due to HIPPA requirements, which protects a patients confidentiality, names and details of their conditions, have not been included. Some are even a conglomerations of common threads that run together that are often relatable.

This book is directed toward females with a vagina and vulva. However, the term woman can be used by anyone who identifies themselves as such. It is written within the framework of penetration/insertion for the purpose of sexual intercourse, tampon use, toys and being able to have an internal exam by a professional. And as we all know, sex itself is a broadly used term that can mean a variety of things in a variety of settings and combinations, not just penetration of a penis in a vagina. The large majority of my experience is with woman that are partnered up with a man, but having a partner is not a prerequisite for the use of the book. The principles can easily be adapted to a single person engaging in solo pleasure, a homosexual/lesbian couple, or as someone who has experienced gender affirmation surgery.

I am also sensitive to the fact that sexual trauma is not an uncommon event. And there are times that is is often left untreated or hiding deep in the recesses of the mind. If at any time in reading the following pages or participating in any suggested assignments, you find yourself struggling with any unwanted feelings, fears or anxiety not yet processed, please seek the assistance from licensed professional specifically trained in this. There are plenty of resources out there to help guide you.

To my dearest mother, Dottie Moran, who has always been my guiding light and my biggest source of inspiration. I am forever grateful for the unwavering love and support you have shown me throughout my life, especially during the times when I felt lost and unsure of myself. You have taught me what it means to be a strong, compassionate, and resilient woman.

As I wrote this book, I couldn't help but think of you and the countless ways you have impacted my life. You have always stood in your power with grace and humility, inspiring me to do the same. You have taught me to be kind and forgiving, even in the face of adversity. Your unwavering faith has been a constant source of comfort and reassurance.

It is because of you that I have found the courage to write about a subject that is often misunderstood and stigmatized. You have shown me that it is possible to talk about difficult topics with empathy and understanding, and I hope to do the same with this book. I dedicate this book to you, my mother, with all my heart. Thank you for being my anchor, my greatest source of love and inspiration as my Mother, my role model, and my friend.

In loving memory and always in my heart
5/15/1927–3/26/2021

There is a beautiful poem by Erin Henson that reads: There is freedom waiting for you, On the breezes of the sky, And you ask, "What if I fall?" Oh but my darling, "What if you fly?"

Table of Contents

Letter to My Readers

Dearest readers,

Are you tired of feeling pain and discomfort during intimacy? Are you tired of feeling like there is something wrong with you and alone in your despair? Do you wish you could unlock your sexual potential and embrace intimacy without fear or discomfort? If so, I have some exciting news for you.

Painful Sex No More is the comprehensive guide to pain-free intimacy and the path to sexual wellness. In its pages, you will find practical tips and advice for exploring your sensuality, cultivating a deeper sense of self-confidence, and experiencing intimacy without pain.

Through my own journey of self-discovery and healing, I have learned that intimacy is about so much more than just physical pleasure. It's about connecting with yourself, your partner, and the world around you in a deeper and more meaningful way. It's about unlocking your full potential as a sexual being and embracing your unique desires and needs.

In this book, I share my personal experiences and insights, as well as the latest research and techniques for overcoming sexual pain and discomfort. Whether you are dealing with a medical condition, recovering from trauma, or simply looking to enhance your sexual wellness, this book has something for everyone.

So if you're ready to take your intimacy and sexual wellness to the next level, I invite you to join me on this journey. Together, we can unlock your full potential and embrace the joy and pleasure of pain-free intimacy.

Thank you for your interest in this book, and I can't wait to hear about your own journey to sexual wellness.

From the heart, Sandi Smith, PT

Foreword

When I first met Sandi at an event, I was leading a few years back, I knew she was special. The calming energy, kindness, empathy, and compassion could be felt from across the room. As I got to know her and her work, she made a true impression on me as both a healer and a friend. I was especially impressed when she shared a bit about how she had successfully worked with many patients on a particular problem that I often see—*pelvic floor dysfunction* and the associated issues that come with the diagnosis.

As an internal medicine physician with a practice that is a blend of traditional medicine along with integrative/functional medicine, I have found that pelvic floor dysfunction is found in 1 in 3 women, and most don't talk about it. And if they do, there is extreme embarrassment and frustration.

Here is an example of what happens when I walk in to see a patient that I see once or twice a year for a physical. Because I am in the minority of docs that spend the time to ask—and even then it is not until the last 5 minutes when sometimes we are already in the hall—they tell me about their lives. That is when

I hear, "*Dr. Lisa, there is one more thing...*" and they spill the beans:

"I leak urine.
I feel dry and itchy down there.
Ever since I can't have sex because it hurts.
I just assume there is nothing you can do but thought I would ask."

Then they add that if I were a male doctor, they wouldn't even mention it. Along with all these symptoms, there usually are a lot of other related issues like anxiety, decreased self-esteem, recurrent UTIs, and urinary incontinence to mention a few.

As a functional medicine doctor, I treat people more naturally and avoid meds whenever possible. Antibiotics and anticholinergics (the class of drugs used to treat incontinence) have a lot of side effects and long-term issues. Often when I provide bioidentical hormones, many symptoms improve, but not all of them. Pelvic floor PT has been able to help fill in many of the gaps.

I have been excited about pelvic floor PT since I first learned about it a few years back. I have seen it help with everything from urinary incontinence to sexual dysfunction to recurrent UTIs. But it can go even further than that because we hold a lot of our experiences and traumas in our bodies and tissue/fascia.

I have a long medical history that includes the removal of an ovary due to leukemia I had as a teen. The associated chemotherapy and procedures such as bone marrow biopsies and injections in my lower spine left scarring. The trauma of the procedures were things that I thought I had processed through meditation, energy work, therapy, and so much more.

And yet, when I had the opportunity to try pelvic floor therapy and fascial release, I found myself releasing negative/traumatic energy. I realized I still had stuck images and emotions of the past and allowed myself to grieve that part of me and all that I had been through. It was so freeing and such a surprise all at the same time! I felt stronger and more open and morecreative after the treatments.

I believe most of us can benefit from this work even without a history of obvious sexual abuse, illness, or other issues. Sandi has developed a novel approach and is able to guide patients in helping themselves whether they decide to proceed with a therapist or do the work at home. She has an incredible level of compassion that comes through in her writing. The stories you will read in the pages that follow will motivate and excite you.

It is no longer necessary for you to try and find the strength to bring this up with your doctor alone. You can follow the recommendations in this book and get started today. When you do decide to discuss it with a professional, you can now feel strong and grounded in your knowledge that this is a real and common condition that responds to pelvic floor PT!

Dr. Lisa Saff Koche, MD
ABAARM, FAAMFM with Spectra Wellness

Introduction

Some may ask, why a book about painful intercourse? The simple answer is this...

It's one of the most common pelvic floor conditions, often left untreated, underdiagnosed, or dismissed. Whether you're a virgin with no sexual experience, a new mommy who's postpartum, a woman on oral contraceptives, a cancer survivor who underwent radiation, or in pre- or post-menopause ... this book is written for you and the myriad of other women, just like you, who are suffering unnecessarily and often in silence. It is geared toward the cisgender woman but the principles can be applied to someone who has undergone gender affirmation surgery.

It's time to remove the shroud of shame that accompanies this topic. It's time to realize that painful intercourse isn't the norm. It isn't something that you just bite the bullet and push through, hoping to put behind you as soon as possible. For all those times you wanted to tell your partner, your doctor, or your best friend, I honor you!

The notion of sharing this with someone is no easy task. It requires some vulnerability, some trust, and some hope that maybe, just maybe, it doesn't have to be this way. Have you ever thought to yourself, If I could only find a guidebook to help me through this difficulty? Well, you're in luck. Think of the content herein as timeless advice from a caring confidant. It's written from a place of compassion and kindness—by someone who truly knows how you feel. Every word was carefully chosen for you. Every photo, diagram, link, and recommendation was chosen for a reason. The flow from chapter to chapter is very much intentional. May you find comfort in my words! May my guidance empower you to discover a better version of yourself! May it lead you down a road to freedom in experiencing the sense of comfort that you've been searching for. And ultimately, may it provide you with the tools to have pain-free intercourse.

How to Use This Book

Though we live in a society of instant gratification, this process isn't going to be instantaneous. It's not a race, it's a journey. The book has been designed to flow like multiple visits to a pelvic-health therapist. At the end of each chapter, you will find real stories from real patients that are 100% unedited. I did provide the questions for them to consider. I wish to thank those of you who took the time to add this personal touch for my readers to hear from you and how this process changed your lives. What I'm offering in this practical manual is the same information that I offer my patients over the course of a plan of care to address painful intercourse. It begins with education. It transitions into movement and breathing. Next comes some self-discovery and reflection. Then, comes the process of completing at-home assignments meant to complement one another. Finally comes ease-of-intimacy and corresponding pleasure. Each chapter should be read in sequence, and time should be taken between chapters to apply the elements and absorb the essence. You can't get to the final destination without taking each individual step. After all, it's rarely the destination that changes us but the journey itself.

There's much to discover if you allow yourself the opportunity to do so. The material ahead will most likely challenge you on multiple levels. The first is most evident, and that's the physical level. However—what's more—I can almost guarantee it will cause you to question your beliefs about sexuality and pleasure. It's important that you respect your own progress and, by all means, take your time. It really is a quest for something better, and this pilgrimage belongs to you alone.

Most often, this condition doesn't come about overnight. It takes time to develop, and it will take time to unravel as well. Consider this process an opportunity to discover a new part of yourself—one that you've never known or somehow lost along the way. Regardless of where you have been, allow this to be the beginning of something exquisite. My wish for you is that you'll find the answers to questions you never considered asking. My hope is that you'll find solutions that make a difference and impact your life in ways you never imagined.

1

What's Your Story?

Do you often feel like you're all alone in dealing with painful intercourse and think that no one else is experiencing this kind of pain? The stories below will assure you that you're NOT alone. An astounding number of women can relate to your story. The American College of Obstetrics and Gynecologists reports that number to be as high as 75 percent. That's right, 75 percent! This condition is probably more common than you ever imagined. Read on and see who you might identify with most.

The Story of the Virgin Bride

It was a picturesque Spring day in the South. The dogwoods were in full bloom, and the azaleas were opening in every shade imaginable. The sky was sapphire blue, and there wasn't a cloud as far as the eyes could see. It was the perfect day for a wedding. The bride was from one of the most prestigious families in Metro Atlanta. The groom was an up-and-coming country singer—a man on the rise. They'd hired the most expensive and sought-after wedding planner, and every detail had been carefully considered. The bride had the gown custom-designed by Monique Lhullier, and it fit like a glove. The wedding party could have been on the cover of Southern Bride magazine.

After over a year of planning, the day had finally arrived. The venue was magical, and the flowers were resplendent. Time seemed to stand still when the virgin bride finally walked down the flower-pedal-covered aisle. The day went off without a hitch. They danced late into the night, and there was magic in the air. Exhausted from the excitement of the day, they waited so long to share, the newlyweds fell into a deep sleep—in each other's arms—only to wake the next day to catch a flight to the ultimate post-nuptial getaway: namely, Bali. The night of consummation had arrived. But soon, her dream turned into a nightmare. The pain was excruciating! No matter what they tried, it was to no avail. How could this happen? She was crushed. No one had prepared them for this. And despite his best efforts, nothing he did would console her. They made the best of the days ahead, but the feelings of disappointment and embarrassment loomed over them like a cirrus cloud.

The Story of the Empty-Nesters

They had been married for thirty-one years and had five amazing children and six precious grandchildren. They couldn't have been more proud of how their family had flourished. The kids were all successful in their chosen fields, and the oldest three were becoming conscientious parents themselves. It was finally time for the youngest son to head off to the college of his dreams on a full scholarship. They'd picked the perfect dorm in an Ivy League school, and the stage was set for the empty nest they had dreamed of settling into. They no longer had to make sure the bedroom door was closed or that they might be overheard during a late night of passion. Yet ... in the months ahead, intimacy became painful. First, it was a little painful, and lubricant helped. But it soon became unbearable. What could be the problem?

The Story of the New Mom

She had waited for what seemed like an eternity to have this baby—featuring numerous in-vitro attempts and years of not being able to get pregnant naturally. Actually, the pregnancy went exceptionally well, and she enjoyed every moment of it. She wanted to deliver the baby naturally with the assistance of a midwife and a doula at a birthing center with the hopes of a water delivery. The labor wasn't as difficult as she had prepared herself for, and everything worked out as planned, except for a moderate-sized vaginal tear, which required stitches. She gave birth to a beautiful baby girl named Isabella.

Her first months as a new mommy were full of surprise and wonder as her baby girl smiled and cooed. She would look into her eyes, and the resultant feelings she experienced were indescribable. Soon, the time came time for her and her husband to reunite in the bedroom for the intimacy they both longed to share again. She was somewhat concerned, but she figured that with plenty of foreplay and the lubricant that had always worked in the past, it would all be okay. But, it wasn't.

The Story of the Dancer

She was a highly successful dancer at The New York City Ballet. She worked tirelessly and spent years in training through her childhood and academic years to enter the profession of her dreams. It was a very difficult journey full of countless hours of practice and numerous injuries. There was no time in her life for anything other than dance. But one day after a show, she met a very special man. Time went on, and they soon became inseparable. The night came when she felt ready to get closer. But wait. This wasn't as easy as she had hoped. Despite his best efforts, he was unable to penetrate. He knew that he was her first, but they both had figured with time and patience, it would eventually work out. Weeks turned into months, and months turned into years. But their love continued to grow. They finally had a long heart-to-heart talk one day and decided that something had to be done.

The Story of the Transgender Awakening

Jonathan was twenty-one years old, and his mother looked across the kitchen table one morning and asked, "Honey, do you think you would be happier as a woman?" Embarrassed and unsettled, he responded quickly, "Well, of course not, Mom. What makes you say that?" The conversation awkwardly ended, and life went on. Jonathan had the perfect Disney wedding followed by a fun-filled honeymoon at the Magic Kingdom. Things seemed smooth at first but with the passage of time, his dysphoria became real. After some time, he started experimenting with cross-dressing. At first, his wife understood but as time marched on, this became a deal-breaker, and the divorce ensued. He continued to live his life cross-dressing, and it seemed to be enough. But one day, he had a dream. He had died and saw himself in a coffin. The family and friends were gathered around, but no one could see Johnathan. He woke up and realized no one could see him because he really wasn't living his life as his true self in the body he was given. This dream was all he needed to push him to make the decision he had been wrestling with. He decided to travel to Baltimore, to see the best plastic surgeon in the US and consulted with him on gender affirmation surgery. The date was set, and the decision was made.

The recovery was grueling and exceptionally painful. But with the help of loved ones, she recovered and began living the life she was meant to live. She finally found the happiness she'd been looking for. The process of preparing her body to live with this physical alteration involved many actions. She began her post-recovery program with the greatest of enthusiasm.

The Story of the Young Widow

She and her husband had been happily married for eleven years. Their lives and their love were written like pages in a fairy tale—filled with romance, travel, a lovely home, a close-knit group of friends, and a large family that lived nearby. But one day on the way to work, he was killed in a tragic car accident. She was crushed beyond measure. No one could have prepared her to be a widow at the age of thirty-two. Life marched on, and time passed ever so slowly, but nine years later, she met someone endearing and fell in love. No one had been close to her in all those years, but there was something very special about him. The time came for them to share their intimacy, and although she was a little nervous, she had no idea this was going to be so painful. How had nine years of not being sexually active changed her body that much?

The Story of the Survivor

Both her mother and her great-grandmother developed endometrial cancer. Hope as she may, she was unable to dodge this MMR gene mutation bullet either. At forty-four, she was diagnosed with stage-two cancer. A complete hysterectomy and radiation was the recommendation of MD Anderson, and the surgery was scheduled. The recovery was difficult but not unbearable—thanks to the care and compassion of her loving husband and two terrific daughters. Day by day, she got stronger and was soon able to return to her active life of tennis, Pilates, and yoga. She knew that it would be some time before she and her husband could share the closeness they once did, but she was patient with the recovery process. She consulted with a pelvic-health physical therapist and soon learned all the lessons necessary to return to sharing the intimacy she once knew.

The Story of the Good Girl

She was raised by extremely conservative parents who weren't very open about their feelings. Her upbringing was strict, and she walked a narrow path to keep everyone happy. They had high expectations for her and her two siblings, and there was always pressure to outperform her classmates. Getting straight A's was the rule of order, and anything less created a great deal of disappointment and a deep sense of failure.

The day that every young girl fears came, and she started her menstrual cycle. Try as she might, she was unable to use tampons like all her friends. Her Mother tried to counsel her, but with much embarrassment and shame, she never did succeed. She felt like she ruined many a family vacation by not being able to fully participate in all the fun. At eighteen, her first visit with a gynecologist was a disaster, as the pain proved unbearable. Her first exam was rescheduled for the following week under anesthesia. She felt like she was broken, and the sense of failure weighed on her like a lead apron.

The Story of "I Just Need a Break"

She had been in a number of serious relationships over the years, and her last one of sixteen years essentially drained her on every level. One day, she looked at herself in the mirror and said, "What happened to Becca? Where did she go? I must go find her!" It was time to take a break from relationships and find her true self again. This was an opportunity to work on reconnecting with her purpose and find out what truly made her happy. It was freedom to take some much-needed time to reflect, relax, and just be. Having reconnected with friends and family, read some fantastic books on self-discovery, and enjoyed a number of hours in the company of a compassionate therapist, she felt empowered to venture out. She met a fantastic guy named Christian, and after a number of months of getting to know one another, it felt like the right time for that magic night. Much to her surprise, however, this break affected her pelvic floor in a way that she hadn't expected. For the first time in her life, she experienced pain while being intimate.

And Now: The Story of YOU

As you can see, painful intercourse comes in a variety of colors. It can occur at any stage of life and for any number of reasons. It doesn't discriminate by age, race, socioeconomics, nationality, or sexual preference. You may ask yourself how something so natural can be so complicated, but the bottom line is that it can be. Whichever story you identify with the most, remember one thing: YOU'RE NOT ALONE! "It's estimated that 46–60 percent of women experience painful intercourse at some time in their lives."[1] The best news of all is that it can be treated and has a very high rate of success. It's actually one of the most successfully treated of all sexual disorders, with the success rates often reaching 100 percent! This book is a guide, full of sage wisdom and practical advice that can be easily understood and implemented. May it provide you with all the tools that you need to find comfort, self-compassion, and happiness.

What exactly is the problem and when was it first discovered?

In 1861, an American gynecologist named Dr. J. Marion Sims described the syndrome known as vaginismus. It was linked to hypersensitivity of the pelvic floor and was commonly considered to be caused by muscular spasms, which prevented vaginal penetration. Sims' answer was surgery, which was later identified as an unnecessary and ineffective procedure. Over time, Sims became the subject of much debate in France, and Vaginismus: A Franco-American Story can be found on PubMed if you would like to read more.

To further complicate this subject matter, the issue has scarcely been discussed until fairly recently. "The Diagnostic and Statistical Manual of Mental Disorders, 5th Edition, (DSM 5)"[2] 2013, classifies vaginismus and the diagnosis of

[1]Glatto AE, Zinner SH, McCormack WMThe Prevalence of Dyspareunia; Obstetrics Gynecology 1970 75: 433-436
[2]The American Psychiatric Association 5th edition; Washington DC 2013
Diagnostic and Statistical Manual of Mental Disorders

dyspareunia under the umbrella of the more expansive category "Genito-Pelvic Pain Penetration Disorder" (GPPPD), and it's grouped into four categories:

1. Primary, in which the patient has never experienced non-painful intercourse;
2. Secondary, in which the patient has previously experienced non-painful intercourse;
3. Global, in which the patient experiences pain with any and all forms of vaginal penetration like a tampon or during a routine gynecological exam; and
4. Situational, in which a patient experiences pain with some types of penetration but not during others.

According to the American College of Gynecologists (ACOG), up to three out of four women experience pain with penetration at some time in their lives. With this in mind, the question remains: Why is this all-too-common condition so poorly understood? It's actually one of the most common conditions regarding the pelvic floor and affects millions of women worldwide. It's often misunderstood by professionals, both in the field of medicine and psychology. It isn't well-presented in medical schools, residency programs, or medical meetings offering continuing education. Its complexity has biological, psychological, and social dimensions. The bottom line here is that this condition is significantly under-researched. There are very few well-controlled studies looking at causes or treatments. As of the writing of this book, there are 448 studies in the category of vaginismus found on PubMed. On the contrary, there are 2731 studies found under the category of erectile dysfunction. The term vaginismus itself isn't well-understood among healthcare providers and often unknown to many women. A related term is dyspareunia, which specifically refers to intercourse. Often, women with this condition can comfortably use tampons and have yearly exams with minimal discomfort. Yet, both of these conditions cause women to experience fear, anxiety, depression, and of course, pain with respect to penetration. These conditions can often lead to unconsummated marriages, sterility, or the separation of a couple.

What causes Vaginismus? And, more importantly ... why is this happening to ME?

We often don't know exactly what causes this condition, as there are many layers to the onion. That being said, having a medical examination before beginning any intervention is always done in order to rule out any underlying pathology. Keep in mind that if there are any underlying medical conditions that need to be treated, the pain will usually be more constant in nature, and not provoked by penetration alone. Regardless, the presence of any of the following conditions is possible, in which case medical treatment is vital:

- Infections like UTIs or yeast infections (i.e., vaginitis)
- The presence of a cyst or fibroids
- Pelvic inflammatory disease (PID)
- Endometriosis
- Cancer
- Pelvic floor prolapse
- Menstrual disorders

- Polycystic ovarian syndrome (PCOS)
- Sexually transmitted diseases (STDs)
- Lichens sclerosis
- Vulvodynia or vestibulodynia
- Eczema or psoriasis

Other possible links which may be physical or non-physical sources:

- Pelvic floor muscle clinching/tightening (most common cause)
- Inadequate foreplay and or insufficient lubrication (second-most common cause)
- A hip injury or fall on the tailbone
- Menopause/hormonal imbalances
- Vaginal atrophy/thinning of the walls
- Oral birth control or other medication side effects
- Previous surgeries such as a hysterectomy or cesarean
- Radiation therapy
- Drug therapies for depression like SSRIs (Selective serotonin reuptake inhibitors)
- Cultural or religious beliefs/upbringing
- A history of sexual abuse
- Mental conditions such as depression or anxiety
- Stress
- Low self-esteem or shyness
- Fear due to lack of sexual experience
- Relationship issues such as unresolved conflicts or lack of trust
- Childbirth and postpartum recovery

- Childhood experiences due to overly rigid parents or inadequate sex education
- Over-reactive or hypersensitive nervous system
- High-intensity training (HIT)/heavy core exercise
- A history of holding the bladder or bowels due to work schedules or not wanting to use public restrooms

As you can see, vaginismus/dyspareunia is a unique condition that may result from a combination of both physical and non-physical causes or may seem to have no cause at all. Whatever the reason, once there has been medical clearance and no other treatment has been recommended, then the journey can begin toward a more satisfying sexual experience and the happiness you have longed for. Are you ready to let go of the pain, the guilt, the shame, and the embarrassment? Of course, you are—or you wouldn't have picked out this book.

So, what are the symptoms exactly?

Consider the following questions:

1. Is initial or deep insertion painful or virtually impossible?
2. Is it difficult to insert tampons or get internal exams?
3. Does fear/anxiety accompany the thought of penetrative sex?
4. Do you feel tightness or muscle spasms in the pelvic area?
5. Do you carry tension or tightness in your hips, abdomen, and/or lower back?

6. Are you able to consciously contract and more importantly relax your pelvic floor muscles (Kegel/reverse Kegel)?
7. Do you feel like your vagina is too tight?
8. Do you have constipation/trouble emptying your bowels or bladder and have to strain to pee?
9. Do you have urinary incontinence (leaking when you sneeze, cough, laugh, lift, and/or exercise)? This could be a sign that your pelvic floor is too tight. A tight muscle is also most likely a weak muscle.

It's my hope that this book will provide you with a full spectrum of solutions and a look at multiple treatment options that complement each other. They are designed to be carried out in the privacy of your home with or without a partner. You will see that there are many spokes to the wheel. There isn't one answer with a one-size-fits-all mentality. The best answer is the one that works for you in your set of unique circumstances. The purpose of this book is to empower you to better understand yourself and your body. The end game is a set of instructions regarding how to achieve-pain free intercourse. May you enjoy the journey to intimacy and more importantly, to a new sense of self.

Real Stories from Real Patients: EC

Would you like to tell the readers a little about yourself?

I'm 25 years old and have been in a long-term relationship for 5 years.

How long have you been dealing with this condition and what other treatments have you tried?

I have had this condition my whole life as far as I know. Since I was a preteen I was never able to use tampons because of the pain I experienced. I always thought it was normal or I was just being a baby so I opted to use pads just to avoid the discomfort. I never tried any treatment because it wasn't until I had tried to have sex for the first time (with my current boyfriend) that I realized the pain I was experiencing was more than just the stereotypical "popping my cherry" or "virgin pain". Luckily I had a very compassionate boyfriend who was patient (and with me for my killer sense of humor instead of my body) and we found ways to enjoy intimacy that didn't include penetration. A few years into our relationship I finally got my first "big girl job" that came with health insurance and I was able to finally go to the OBGYN to figure out what was going on. That's when she recommended pelvic floor physical therapy.

Did you have a positive outcome/were you pleased with the results and why?

I had an amazing outcome and I can't be more happy with my results. I am able to have sex and use tampons with very minimal pain. The only time it is painful to have sex now is if I go a few days without and haven't kept up with my stretches. But after a minute or two of slowly allowing the penetration to happen, the pain goes away.

Did you find the material/assignments easy to understand?

Yes, the diagrams given were super helpful and Sandi did a great job of demonstrating and explaining everything in detail.

Did you find the assignments easy to implement? Why or why not?

Yes, the stretches were relaxing and functional so it was easy to add to the end of a workout or even right before bed to wind down.

What were your biggest challenges and why?

My biggest challenge was actually overcoming the shame and guilt of not being able to have sex with my partner. As a woman, not being able to physically do what my body was made to handle felt so shameful. However, Sandi not only helped me overcome the physical obstacles but the mental ones too. Finally understanding what was going wrong and working toward fixing it gave me so much more confidence and I am no longer ashamed to talk about my struggle with vaginismus, whereas before, my boyfriend was the only one who knew we weren't having sex.

What did you find was the easiest thing to do and why?

The stretches and breathing exercises were the easiest to do. As I said earlier, they were relaxing and easy to implement into my lifestyle and workout routine.

Would you recommend this treatment plan to others?

Absolutely. I've already recommended it to a few people in my life that have mentioned sex hurts sometimes.

How long did it take to start seeing results?

My treatment took about 6 months I believe but I was seeing results as soon as I started using the dilators. I wasn't even able to handle the smallest one at first but within 3 months I could use the larger sizes.

Would you like to add anything to help the readers better understand the process and what it takes to be successful?

The biggest key to success in my experience is using dilators and getting over the mental blocks. I was so close to giving up because I was still experiencing some discomfort with the dilators and was telling myself the pain is always going to be there. But one night I randomly decided to just give sex a try and boom! It happened. Take it slow. Relax. And try to enjoy the moment rather than looking at sex as a giant obstacle you have to tackle and get through. You can get through it, you just have to put in the work.

2

How Can Physical Therapy Help?

Are you wondering why the silence is finally being broken ... at least a bit? Due to social media and more medical professionals getting on board with this once-taboo subject matter, painful intercourse is finally being talked about. The days of being told by a doctor it's all in your head, just drink a glass of wine, or take some Advil are long gone ... at least I hope they are. Physical therapy is really on the front line in spreading the good news and shedding some much-needed light on a condition that was once in the dark.

The field of physical therapy was started in the US in 1921 by Mary McMillian, who was a trailblazer—now considered the mother of physical therapy. Most people are familiar with what a physical therapist does and what they might treat. Yet, comparatively, few realize there is a specialty called pelvic health. Fast forward to 1977 when Elizabeth Nobel founded the Academy of Pelvic Health Physical Therapy with the American Physical Therapy Association (formally the Section on Women's Health). Today, this organization has more than 3900+ physical therapists, physical therapy assistants, and students. This is a post-graduate specialty track and includes the treatment of women, men, and children with pelvic floor disorders.

The question remains: What does a PT do and how can this help me? The bottom line is that a PT is the most skilled professional available to address issues that surround the pelvic floor. You might ask, what exactly is a pelvic floor? Within the female pelvis, this band of muscles and connective tissue acts like a hammock or sling to support and suspend the uterus, fallopian tubes, ovaries, bladder, and bowels. Within the male pelvis, they support the bladder and bowels and key play a role in sexual function. They are located vertically between the pubic bone and the tailbone and horizontally between the two sitting bones. Like any other muscle, they need to be dynamic with the ability to contract and relax as needed.

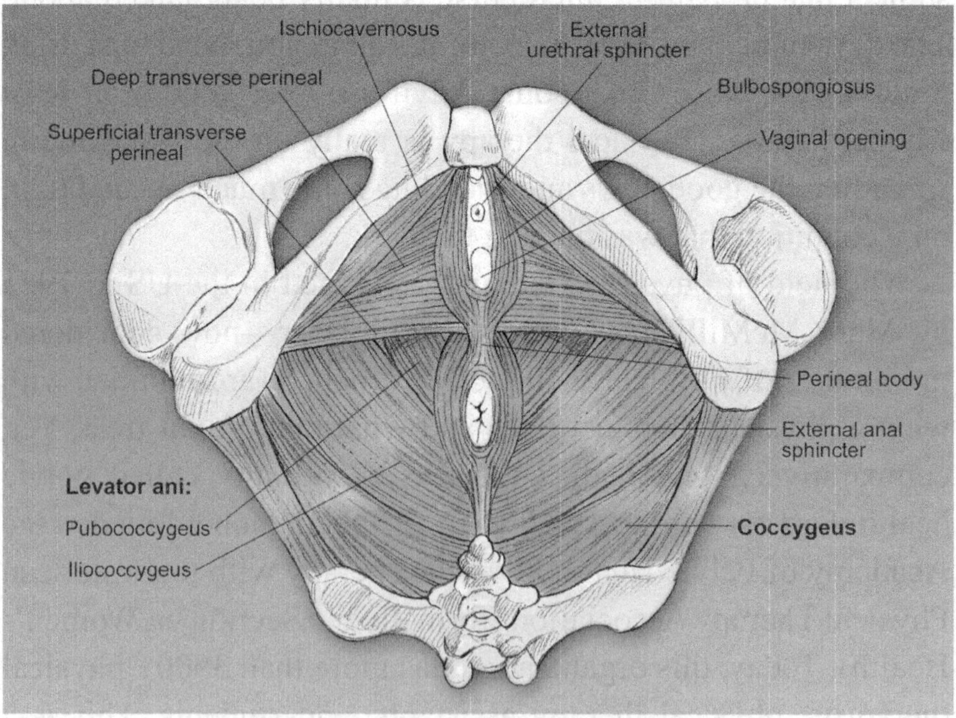

So, what happens to the pelvic floor when intercourse is painful due to vaginismus? Simply put, the muscles become too tight or overactive, thus creating increased tension. In essence, the sling has become too short or taut, making insertion painful, if not impossible. This can lead to poor blood flow and nerve irritation, often making them tender and painful or sensitive to touch. The best news of all is that these muscles can and do lengthen. With the proper amount of stretching, directed in the right way, they adapt and find a new length that allows penetration to occur with comfort and ease.

What to Expect If You See a PT

First of all, it's important to know that most states do allow a patient to see a PT without a referral from a doctor. Although your insurance may require it, oftentimes this isn't the case, and you can consult independently. Some practices do accept insurance payment and others are "cash-based." You'll need to call your provider of choice to see what the arrangement is. To find a PT near you, the best resources are:

1. The American Physical Therapy Association (APTA) at www.apta.org – Choose "Find a Physical Therapist" under the specialty of Women's Health.
2. You can also search www.pelvicrehab.com for the Herman and Wallace practitioners directory.

Regardless of who you see or where you go, the therapist will always have an intake procedure to begin the process. This is basic information about your health and your condition. This gives the practitioner a starting point from which to begin to understand you. All PTs follow the SOAP format:

Part 1-Subjective: This entails an extensive interview that allows the therapist to ask all the important questions to get to know you and your condition. This follows a non-judgmental format that allows you to open up and share all your concerns. This is the time you get to know each other and begin to develop a trusting relationship; a relationship based on respect and dignity. In this environment, there is no such thing as TMI (too much information). This is your opportunity to say all the things that you probably find too uncomfortable to talk with anyone else about. This time is pivotal and of paramount importance, for it provides a framework from which to begin.

Part 2-Objective: This is the physical part of the evaluation that usually begins with a basic orthopedic screening looking at the range of motion, strength, posture/alignment, and palpation. Palpation identifies tightness or tenderness in the muscles of the hips, lower back, and abdomen by means of touch and varied pressure. Beyond this, a pelvic specialist is skilled in performing an internal exam. But keep in mind that this may or may not occur on the first visit. This often depends on the complexity of the condition and if time allows. A speculum isn't used like in a gynecologist's office. A gloved finger is used to assess the tissue around the vaginal opening (the more superficial muscles) and inside the vaginal canal (the deeper muscles). This is always first done with verbal/informed and written consent and always takes the patient's comfort level into account. You will remain professionally draped at all times. The main purpose of this part of the exam is to identify the structures that may be causing pain with penetration. This can be either superficial muscles that are surrounding the opening and/or deeper structures within the canal.

Part 3-The Assessment: Here, the therapist reports back to you what the clinical findings were. This is done in a fashion that is easily understood, using terminology that is designed to facilitate patient understanding. It most often involves patient education regarding the anatomy of the pelvis/pelvic floor and possible contributing factors. This is the time to ask questions and put your mind at ease. Our role as educators has never been more important than it is with respect to treating the pelvic floor. Understanding is key, and as the adage goes, knowledge is power. We want to empower you!

Part 4-The Plan: A plan of care is established. This first informs the patient how many visits to expect. It then describes the methods of treatment that will be used to address the clinical findings and what the expected outcome or prognosis is. Some of the most common methods of treatment include patient education/self-care instructions, manual therapy/hands-on techniques (both externally and internally), therapeutic exercises for flexibility and strength, neuromuscular reeducation to help connect the mind and the body, and modalities like electrical stimulation, dry needling, biofeedback, heat, and ice.

The Importance of the Home Program and Your Part

It's important to understand that this is a team effort. The success of the treatment relies a great deal on following through on the suggested recommendations. One of the most important assignments will be your home program. This is often assigned on the first visit if time allows. Our biggest line of defense most often consists of stretches that are designed to increase flexibility in the hips and low back, which are closely related to the pelvic floor. Chapter 4 will be dedicated to this—teaching you phases one, two, and three of the home program.

Self-Care Strategies

Our second line of defense is the recommendation of self-care strategies, which often begin with deep breathing designed to relax the pelvic floor muscles and the central nervous system. Chapter 6 will be devoted to this. Here, you will be given the tools to address many of the issues that may be contributing to this condition. These tools will empower you to take control of your body and your condition, ushering in a successful outcome and the ultimate achievement of pain-free intercourse.

Real Stories from Real Patients: KM

Would you like to tell the readers a little about yourself?

Female, 28 years old, most treatment occurring from age 25–27, found Sandi through a gynecologist recommendation.

How long have you been dealing with this condition and what other treatments have you tried?

I have primary vaginismus, so I first noticed the issue when trying to use a tampon and experienced extreme pain when attempting to insert even the smallest size. Eventually, the problem got in the way of my dating life in addition to not being able to swim or do activities without fear of my pad leaking. Some gynecologists didn't know how to deal with it and gave poor advice or wrote it off as being in my head. One gynecologist immediately believed me and committed to doing everything possible to help me. After a hymenectomy that fixed my microperforated hymen, we discovered that vulvodynia was an issue as she could still barely touch me. I was sent to pelvic PT to work on the muscular tissues as well as desensitize the nerves. After a while, I plateaued because the nerve pain continually made the muscles tighten during manual and dilator therapy. I then did Botox injections (unsuccessful for me) and trigger point injections with a numbing solution followed by an immediate PT appointment to make manual therapy only feel like pressure instead of also having pain. Sandi was also able to do dry needling around that time which resulted in my greatest success as she got the superficial and deep muscles to relax. She was able to bypass any pain with penetration and the muscles tightening reflexively to that pain. From there, I have been able to maintain my results with at-home exercises and dilator therapy. I still have to use lidocaine for larger dilators to make sure the pain doesn't cause the muscles to contract, but I never even thought my body would be able to accommodate the last two sizes.

Did you have a positive outcome/were you pleased with the results and why?

I was very pleased with my results. I came to Sandi unable to get anything more than the first digit of a pinky finger in me to being halfway through my dilator set in the first few months of working with her. After the dry needling, I made it all the way to the largest dilator. It took time, patience, and a lot of hard work, but I felt like Sandi gave me my life back. I was able to use tampons and feel like I could enter the dating pool again when I was ready instead of feeling like I had to avoid it because of this condition.

Did you find the material/assignments easy to understand?

I loved all the baby steps, clear instructions, and variety of assignments/exercises provided. They were easy to follow and very helpful.

Did you find the assignments easy to implement? Why or why not?

Making time for them can be difficult, especially if you have roommates. Once you create a schedule and also remember that a little work is better than no work at all, it's much easier to turn it into a habit and be successful in treatment.

What were your biggest challenges and why?

My first two PT appointments were very painful as the superficial muscles were very tight. She didn't even do any penetration as a result and had to exclusively work through that first. I almost felt like I didn't want to go back and put myself through that pain twice a week, but I also knew it was the only way to get better and that I would have to do PT eventually. Not going back would just delay the inevitable and prolong my treatment process. After a couple of appointments, the pain wasn't as bad plus I understood what I was feeling and why. (Burning, stinging, pressure, muscle spasms, soreness, etc.)

What did you find was the easiest thing to do and why?

The breathing exercises and just getting acquainted with my own body were the easiest for me as they didn't cause any pain or anxiety. While some patients are uncomfortable with their bodies when beginning, this was not the case for me. I simply didn't know the anatomy and muscles well enough to understand what was going on. Doing that resulted in me being much more comfortable using the dilators and seeing gynecologists as I understood my body more.

Would you recommend this treatment plan to others?

I 100% would recommend this plan. No other treatments worked or worked on their own without pelvic PT. I had tried dilators before going to PT, and I couldn't even get the smallest size in on my own. It's best to work with a professional who knows these conditions and the anatomy to help you understand what is going on.

How long did it take to start seeing results?

I started to see results immediately in even just the reduction of pain with sitting and wearing jeans. I was able to graduate to the next dilator size, go from one finger to two, and have fingers go in deeper very frequently throughout treatment which was encouraging to see.

Would you like to add anything to help the readers better understand the process and what it takes to be successful?

I will not lie: it will hurt and be frustrating at times. But this is like working out to lose weight or gain muscle as it will not happen overnight and would be unrealistic to expect instant results. You have to put in the time and effort and follow the instructions to see results. Hiring a personal trainer you see once a week will not help if you don't exercise on your own or follow their instructions for your diet. Pelvic PT is the same way as you won't see results or will have very slow results if you don't consistently show up to your appointments or do the work at home. The pain DOES get better over time. Before you know it, that dilator that looked intimidating now easily fits inside you with no pain. If you're working hard but still plateau at some point, that's okay. It doesn't mean that's the end of it for you but rather you need a different tool or approach to heal the remainder of the muscle/nerve issues. If you're in home maintenance mode or having to take a break from appointments for any reason, make sure to not forget about regularly doing the at-home exercises so you don't lose some of that hard-earned progress.

3

The Interconnectedness of All Things

What the heck is the pelvic floor, and why don't I know more about this?

After all, we live in a society that's very open-minded about sex and sexuality. We see it in advertisements, music videos, and movies—on TV and social media. We read about it in books, blogs, and magazines. But somehow there has been a system breakdown in teaching people about their bodies—specifically, the pelvic floor. Most people don't even know that they have a pelvic floor. Sadly, it isn't something that's well taught in our educational system. Sex education in our schools is centered around the menstrual cycle, abstinence, and how to prevent pregnancies/STDs. It's often embarrassing for parents to talk about this with their kids. Home really is the best and healthiest place to learn about this all-important subject. Just starting with teaching boys and girls the proper names for body parts is a great beginning. It's high time to take the embarrassment out of calling a penis a penis and a vagina a vagina. The pelvic floor is also not a typical topic of conversation among friends over coffee or during happy hour. And, to make matters worse, it isn't even well-covered in most of our best medical schools. There is actually a grassroots non-profit organization called Tight Lipped whose mission is to "fight for a world where those with these conditions are diagnosed correctly, treated effectively, and given compassionate care." They can be found at www.tightlipped.org. They offer a podcast and an 80-page zine including art, poetry, and prose from over 50 contributors. Recently they have started working with residency programs to help OB/GYNs better understand the complexities of this field of study. A portion of the proceeds from this book will be donated to Tightlipped org. to support them in their efforts to support women just like you. All that being said, this book (and others like it) are finally bringing this information to the forefront. It's about time! The bottom line is that until there is a problem "down there," no one even tends to think about what's "down there." So, what is "down there" anyway?

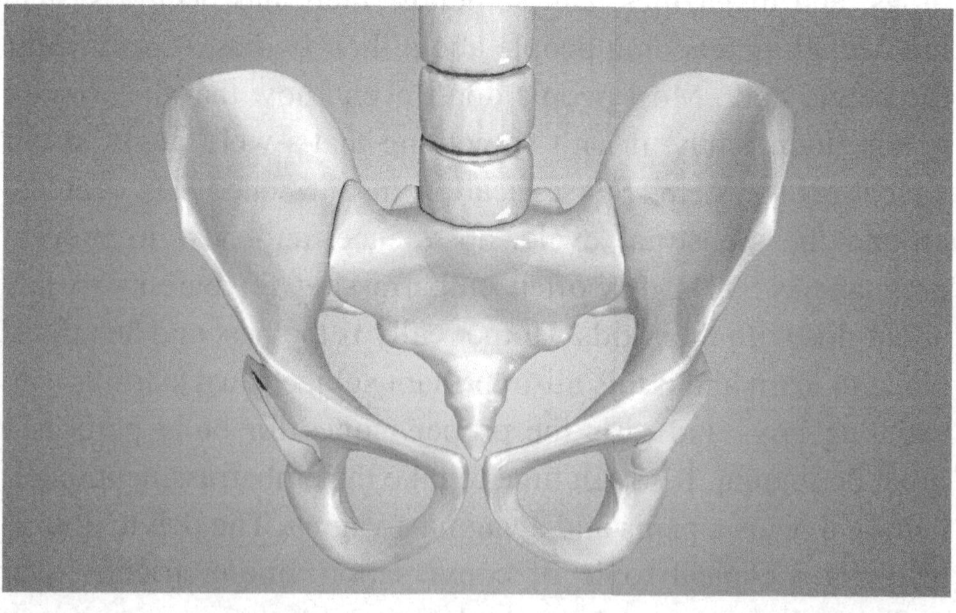

First of all, let's look at what is referred to as the pelvic bowl:

As you can see, the pelvic bowl consists of two half pelvises, which attach to the spine at the sacrum and the legs at the hip joints. When you think about this, it's actually a very complex structure that provides both stability and mobility. It's the connection of the upper torso to the lower legs. It provides attachments for some of the strongest and largest muscles in the body. But what's inside the bowl? The pelvis is the boney structure that contains all of the organs of our urogenital systems: which in the female pelvis consists of the uterus and cervix, the fallopian tubes and ovaries, the bladder and urethra, and the vagina. And it contains the bottom of our digestive system, the sigmoid colon/rectum. So, why is this important to know and understand? Think of the three Ps: All these structures play some role in our basic biological functions of peeing, pooping, and procreating. Again, it's not always something we're comfortable discussing with others, but it is something you may want to keep a watchful eye on and have some knowledge about.

The Interconnectedness of All Things

In the classic model of pelvic physical therapy, the "canister" is often used to describe the connection between the diaphragm (or the top of the canister) and the pelvic floor (the bottom of the canister). It's used as an illustration to provide a platform from which to consider pressures and how these pressures affect the entire system. Understanding this concept of pressure is key and will be further explained.

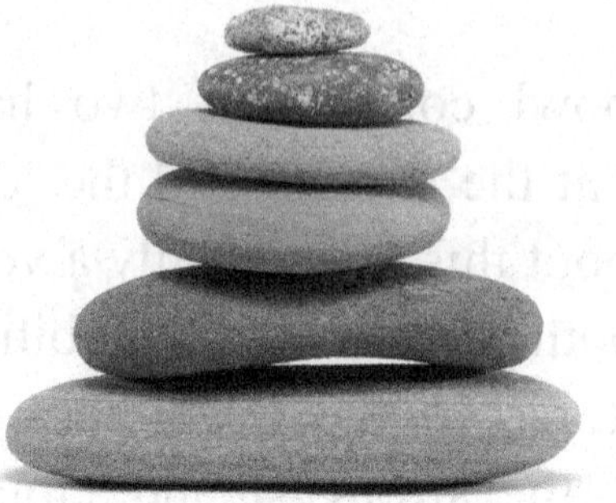

I'd like to expand upon this model and use a Rock Carin to introduce a new illustration.

These (man-made) stacked stones have appeared countless times throughout history. You may have even seen one yourself on one of your own journeys. The name originates from a Scottish Gaelic term that means, "a heap of stones." They're often used to mark trails for navigation or routes of safety. At one time, they were used to mark the land, long before lighthouses. But, dating rock Carins is nearly impossible so, archaeologists have no way of knowing when the earliest stacks were built.

The 5 Rocks of the Pelvic Cairn

Brain
Throat
Heart
Diaphragm
Pelvic Floor

The Brain

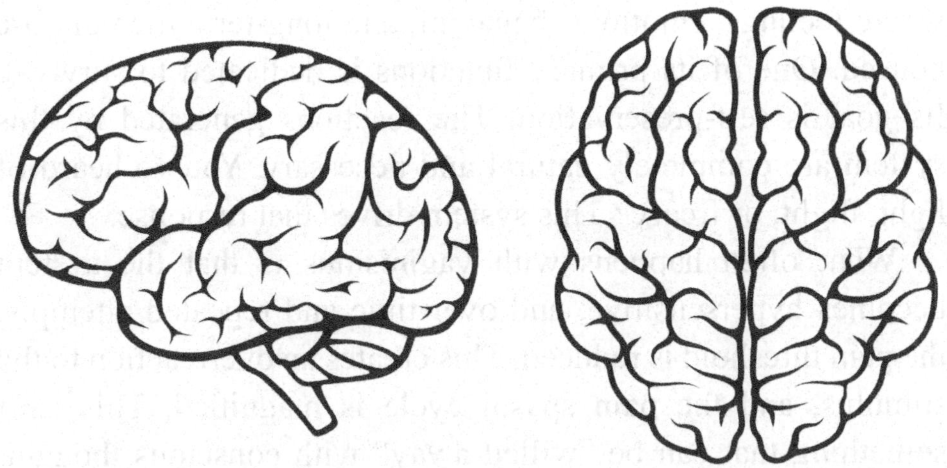

The most common symptom of vaginismus, of course, is pain. In February of 2022, the American Physical Therapy Association Academy of Pelvic Health Physical Therapy presented a webinar by Dr. Bert Messnlink, MD, a renowned and forward-thinking urologist and sexologist in Holland. The title was "You Need the Brain to Treat Pain." In it, he stated, "Pain is a spontaneous response to a perceived treat that promotes healing ... but pain isn't the enemy and hurt doesn't mean harm."

One of the common misconceptions is often that women with this condition don't want to be intimate or engage in sexual activity. This simply isn't true! The response to penetration is completely involuntary and a natural protective pain response. With repeated attempts, the situation only gets worse and soon the brain subconsciously associates penetration with pain. This often leads to stinging and burning as the central nervous system becomes over-activated. The part of the brain that gets overstimulated is referred to as the limbic system, which is controlled by the autonomic nervous system. It's where feelings, emotions, behavior, and long-term memory are housed. One of its primary functions is dedicated to survival. Its goal is self-preservation. The reactions generated by this system are completely natural and necessary. You've heard of fight, flight, or freeze? This system drives that response.

What often happens with vaginismus is that the system becomes hypersensitive, and over time and repeated attempts, the pain threshold is reduced. This creates an overreaction to the stimulus, and the pain spasm cycle is magnified. This isn't something that can be "willed away" with conscious thought. Most importantly, it isn't a woman's fault! This is the ultimate example of the mind-body connection. This can quickly lead to feelings of inadequacy, guilt, shame, anxiety, and embarrassment. This perfect storm is slowly turning into a hurricane of catastrophic dimensions. Over time, the desire for intimacy fades to black ... and the darkness can be overwhelming.

The Throat/Voice

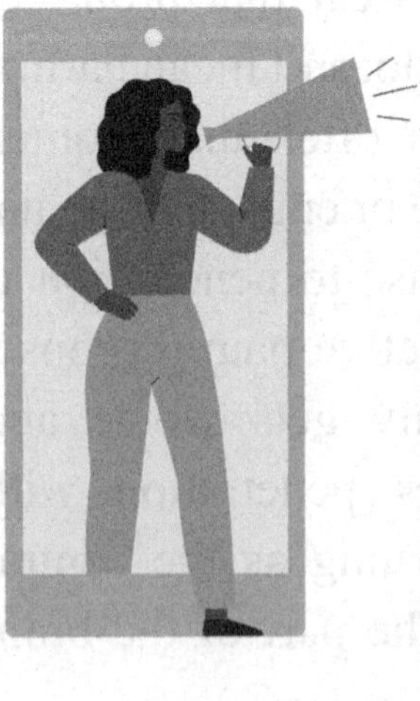

Anyone dealing with this condition knows how difficult it's to discuss it with others. However, keeping it a secret is no longer necessary. It's time to find your voice and tell your doctor, your partner, your friend, and/or your therapist. It's time to remove the stigma and shine the light on something that can often be easily remedied. It's no longer necessary to hide behind the wall of shame that often accompanies this. There isn't anything wrong with you! Once you start talking about it, you'll quickly find out that you're not alone and something can be done about this condition. There is help out there. You just have to find the right resources and take one step at a time.

Today, more and more women are finding their voice, and it's creating a seismic shift in our collective consciousness. Change is in the air, and it's palpable. We're building a bridge from the old paradigm to something new and better, and it's nothing short of revolutionary.

For far too long, the masculine has held dominion over our world. But now, we're seeing a true rising up of the divine feminine, and it's a force to be reckoned with. We're reclaiming our power, our voice, and our rightful place in the world. And we're doing it together, in solidarity and sisterhood.

As we weave this new tapestry, we're creating a world that's more compassionate, more nurturing, and more in tune with our deepest desires and needs. It's a world where women are celebrated and valued, and where the balance between the masculine and feminine is finally being restored.

So let us continue to raise our voices, to stand up for what we believe in, and to create the world we know is possible. Together, we are unstoppable! Check out the Facebook Evolving Sisters Network group for some inspiration. Kenlyn Kolleen has some inspiring messages and great resources as an empowerment leader and spiritual business mentor. You can also find her insightful messages and videos on U-tube under Kenlyn Kolleen.

The Heart

There's so much advancement in the field of medicine these days. It seems we're hitting critical mass in understanding the human body and its complexities. One fascinating discovery made in recent history was the connection between the brain and the heart.

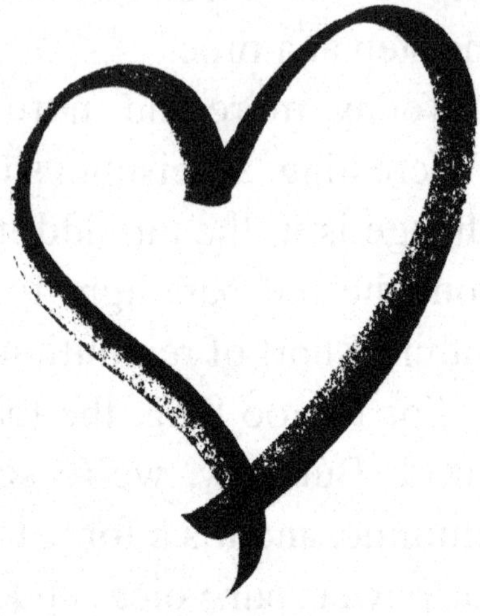

As a result, there's a whole new field of study called neuro-cardiology. In 1991, Dr. J. Andrew Armour discovered that the heart has a "little brain" with approximately 40,000 neurons. It's been identified that the heart is the most powerful source of electromagnetic energy in the human body, producing the largest rhythmic electromagnetic field of any organ. Its electromagnetic field is sixty times greater in

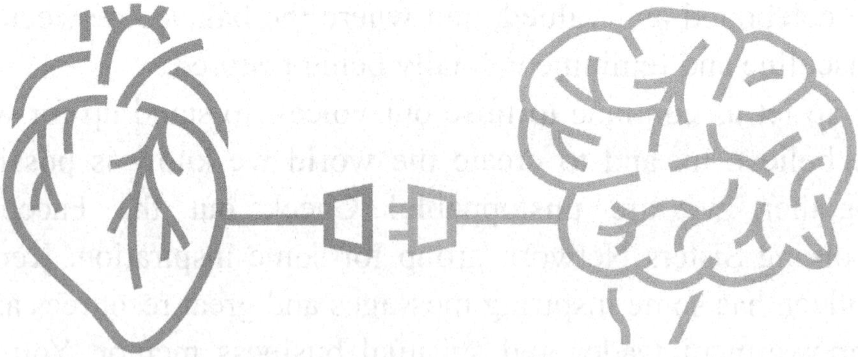

amplitude than that generated by the brain. It's been suggested that the electric field is somewhere between five and eight feet beyond the body. Your heart enters the room before you do! That "little brain" in the heart often "feels" things before our brain can translate. The heart actually sends more information to the brain than the brain sends to the heart. If you're interested in finding out more about this subject, I suggest you explore, HeartMath Institute, located in Boulder Creek, California. Since 1991, this non-profit organization has stayed true to its mission of helping people bring their physical and emotional systems into balanced alignment with their heart's intuitive guidance. They're committed to "Awakening the Heart of Humanity." This company provides scientifically-validated technology that activates the intelligence and power of the heart to dramatically reduce stress while empowering health, performance, and behavioral change. In 2020, they released The HeartMath Experience, www.experience.hearthmath.com. This FREE gift is designed to unlock your heart's natural intuitive guidance, help you better manage stressful emotions, and increase resilience. Here you will find nine ten-minute downloadable PDFs full of compelling content. If you like podcasts, you can also listen to HeartMath's Add Heart with Dr. Deborah Rozman, the president, and CEO.

All that being said, always remember and never forget: follow your heart; it will never lead you astray!!!

The Diaphragm

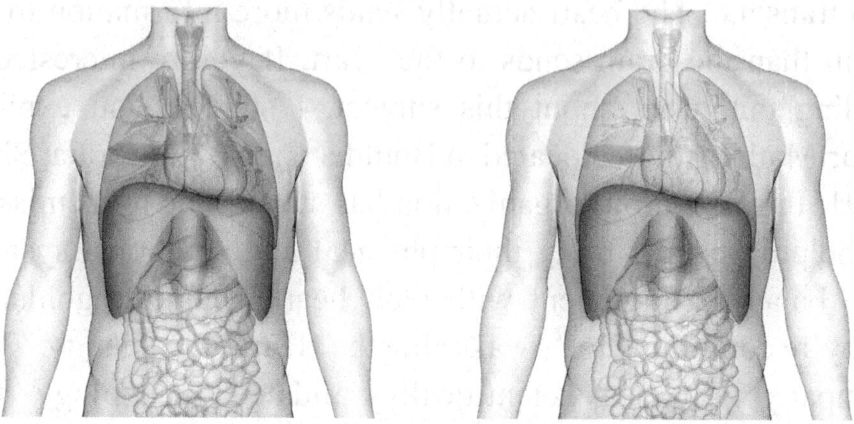

This is the muscle we use every day, often with minimal awareness. It's a thin muscle that sits at the base of the chest and separates the chest from the abdomen. When it contracts, you inhale, which creates a negative pressure to encourage airflow into the lungs. Afterward, the diaphragm relaxes and moves toward the head and creates positive pressure to expel air from the lungs.

We do this approximately 16,000–22,000 times per day, every day.

So, what's the connection to the pelvic floor?

Magically these two sets of muscles mirror one another. As we breathe in, the diaphragm and the pelvic floor descend toward the floor. When we exhale, they ascend toward the head. This concept will come in handy when you learn about reverse Kegels, a key concept to pelvic floor relaxation. The set of muscles between these two structures is commonly called "the core." This is no longer described as a specific structure but rather an interdependent system that provides stability and strength for optimal movement. It's made up of 29+ muscles and described as a muscular box. This understanding will come in handy when you learn to do your own abdominal massage for relaxation and tension release.

The Base Rock of This Cairn: The Pelvic Floor

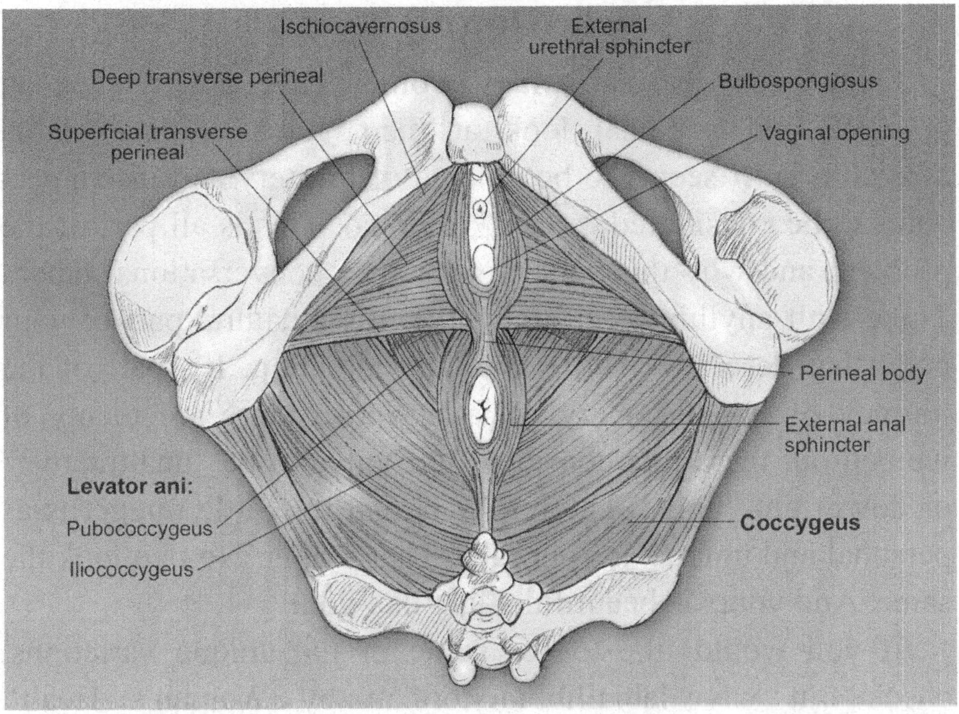

The condition of vaginismus is most often associated with the sling of muscles that supports all of this ... the mysterious pelvic floor. As you can see in the above illustration, this is a rather complex set of muscles, and it serves a vital role. For a variety of reasons, this set of muscles can become tightened or shortened resulting in a hypertonic or state of overactivity. In physical therapy, we address this overactivity with stretches, manual therapy, and reeducation. This now opens the door to all you need to know to address your condition. May your journey be a beautiful one full of surprises and success. May you connect to a part of yourself that you may not have known was there or reconnect to a part of yourself you forgot. Whatever happens, enjoy the journey, and use this pelvic cairn to guide you along the way!

Hello Down There!

Okay, let's get real. Many women have never taken an up-close and personal look at their vulva or inner labia area/clitoris. It seems to be an area of mystery and disconnect and can be considered "weird" to do so. This is all part of the problem and why this subject remains a conversational taboo. There isn't anything weird about it. It's a natural part of your body that deserves a little love and attention. It's part of the journey of self-discovery. What's worse, there are plenty of women out there that consider their vulva to be "unattractive" or downright "ugly." The reality is that this little nugget is as personal and unique as your face. That's right. No two look the same. And yours is beautiful—just like you!

If you would like to see some of the unique variations, check out www.labiallibbrary.org.au by Woman's Health Victoria. These are real women in real photos that haven't been enhanced or photoshopped. And yes, I give you permission to look. It's perfectly okay! It's powerful seeing that there really is no "normal" and certainly no "perfect" labia ... that is, except for yours!

Many of the photos that appear in print are airbrushed to have that "perfect" appearance. And if you consider what you might view in pornography, the porn stars themselves have often been surgically altered or enhanced. Or maybe they just have the "look" the producer was interested in capturing.

Comparing yourself to anything you see in print or in film is self-defeating. We as women have to move beyond this and unite in healing this collective wound. So, take a moment and introduce yourself to a part of your body that you may not know very well. Find some privacy, grab a mirror, and take some time to acquaint yourself with this very special and unique aspect of yourself.

Learn to accept the way it looks in all its oneness and beauty. In all likelihood, it has its asymmetries, its own unique and particular color, and its individual shape and size. It's yours and yours alone. Revel in its beauty!!!

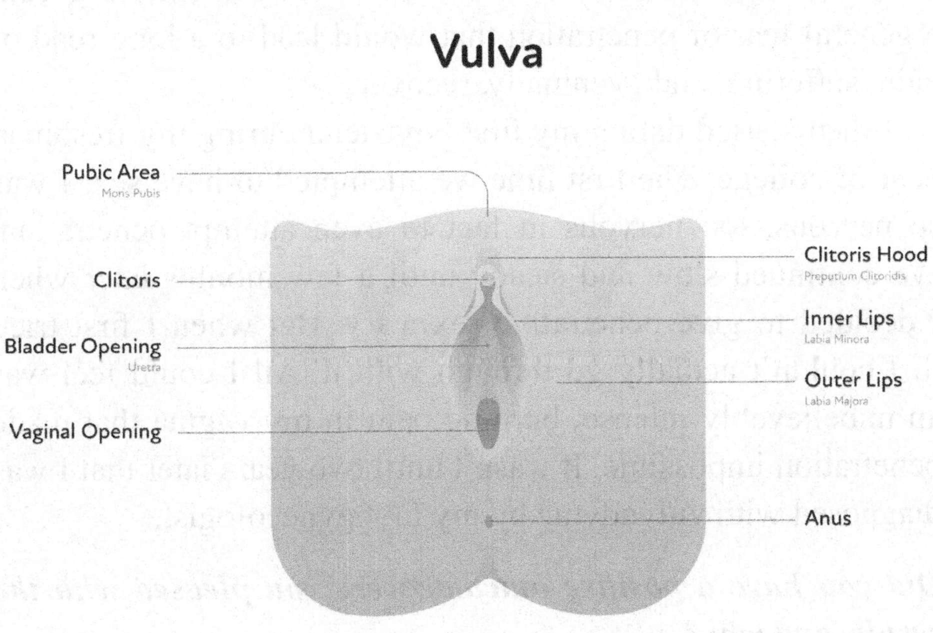

Real Stories from Real Patients: OL

Would you like to tell the readers a little about yourself?

Hello! My name is Olivia. I'm 25 years old and I've been working with Sandi, the book's author, to help with my journey to pain-free sex.

How long have you been dealing with this condition and what other treatments have you tried?

I have been dealing with vaginismus for as long as I can remember. When I was in high school, I was not yet sexually active, but I did have a lot of anxiety and fear around using tampons. Little did I realize at the time that I was suffering from a general fear of penetration that would lead to a long road of pain, suffering, and eventually, recovery.

I then started dating my first boyfriend during my freshman year of college. The first time we attempted to have sex, I was so nervous, too nervous in fact to even attempt penetration. We continued slow and steady until a few months later when I decided to give penetrative sex a try. But when I first tried it, I couldn't actually go through with it. All I could feel was an unbelievably intense, burning pain in my vagina that made penetration impossible. It wasn't until two years later that I was diagnosed with vulvodynia by my first gynecologist.

Did you have a positive outcome/were you pleased with the results and why?

Over the next 5 years, I had attempted every possible treatment I could to cure my condition. My first gynecologist tried to just have me use dilators, but it had very little success. I then decided to switch to a specialist in the area for dealing with female pelvic pain. She had me on gabapentin, testosterone, and estrogen creams, and encouraged me to seek out pelvic floor therapy. It was with that recommendation that my road to recovery had begun.

After I had received a recommendation for physical therapy, I began seeing Sandi to help work my pelvic floor. In all honesty, I was a bit skeptical that the therapy would work. After 5 years of nothing but disappointing results from other forms of treatment, I had it in the back of my mind that I was never going to be able to have sex, let alone pain-free sex. It was a challenging two years I spent working to relax my pelvic floor in therapy and committing to doing exercises often. But after the two long years and a long journey of hard physical work and self-discovery, it finally happened. I was able to have sex! How was this possible?

Did you find the material/assignments easy to understand?

Working with my pelvic floor seemed daunting at first and I didn't see how the therapy would really change anything. As I continued, I still felt frequent pain using the dilators and doing my exercises during sessions. But then, eventually, I started to notice that the pain was becoming less and less. It was difficult to notice, but I was gradually making more and more progress each time I worked on my pelvic floor. I went from not being able to handle one finger, to being able to handle two, then the dilator, then the largest dilators, and it all just naturally worked itself out over time. It was as if my body was working in the background to relax my pelvic floor and feel more calm about putting something into my vagina. And I was finally able to see the results!

Did you find the assignments easy to implement? Why or why not?

The assignments were difficult to stick to at the time. The biggest obstacle for me was the fact that I was in a long-distance relationship, and an unhappy one at that. I wasn't very motivated to implement my exercises and stretches because it felt like I wasn't doing this for a man that I loved and cared about. It felt more like a chore. But my outlook began to change to a more positive one after I ended that relationship and found myself in a new one with a partner I felt much more close and attracted to. Being in a happy relationship had now given me the motivation to work toward the goal, which was pain-free sex. I felt now like there was a light at the end of the tunnel.

What were your biggest challenges and why?

I didn't realize it at the time, but I believe the biggest challenge to my recovery and what hindered me from it was what I felt on the inside. When I started physical therapy, I was still with my first boyfriend, who, in all honesty, from the very beginning, I was not very attracted to. He was a nice guy, but I felt deep down inside as though something was wrong with me because my body just tensed up and did not want him inside of me. The biggest challenge was learning to listen to my body. It was telling me that I wasn't safe, that this wasn't the person I wanted to have such an intimate experience with. After I finally gathered enough courage to end that relationship, I pursued one with a different man, one who made me feel safe and comfortable and I had a connection with, and *most importantly*, whom I was attracted to.

What did you find was the easiest thing to do and why?

The journey to curing my vaginismus was helped not just by my own desire to overcome it, but also by being with a partner who loved me, cared for me, was patient and always by my side, and who I felt a natural desire for. In retrospect, I should have been listening to what my body was telling me about my relationship all along.

Would you recommend this treatment plan to others?

I would highly recommend that any woman suffering from painful intercourse try this treatment plan. It sounds all physical at first, but there really is more to the therapy than just that. By working through pelvic floor therapy, you learn that it's not just physical, but also mental. You learn that your pelvic floor isn't just operating on its own, but rather in symbiosis with the rest of your body, and it all stems from your mental state and your own sense of security. I will never forget the process that led me here, because it taught me more about myself than any other treatment had.

How long did it take to start seeing results?

Ladies, if you are struggling with the same thing I was, I want you to take a step back and really listen to your body. Re-evaluate your life, your relationships, and your sense of self. Becoming self-aware and more confident will help you realize why sex is so anxiety-inducing for you and what you can do to stop your body from having this mental block. Sex can be scary and painful, but it shouldn't be. Having a loving, supportive partner helps so much, as does knowing what you want and feeling confident in yourself. Just remember that there is a light at the end of the tunnel.

4

Let's Get Busy!

My aim is to keep this book short and sweet with the reward of a delightful ending of pain-free intercourse. That being said, hopefully, you have learned a thing or two about your body and feel that by following the guidance in this book, you CAN overcome your pain. After all, these methods are tried and true and have worked on countless women just like you.

This chapter marks the beginning of the instructional manual, which is based on four tenets:

1. The home exercise program: Phase 1, 2, and 3 stretches
2. Relaxation/down training
3. Self-care strategies
4. Fulfillment/Enjoyment

Tenet 1: The Importance of the Home Program

No matter what kind of physical therapist you see or what musculoskeletal concern you may have, I can almost guarantee you one thing: you will be assigned a home program. It isn't uncommon for patients with Vaginismus to have tight hips and/or tight lower back muscles. Let's face it: tight hips and low back are all too common. It's only to be expected, surfing and scrolling our way through the information age. It's even been said that sitting is the new smoking. Our bodies are meant to move! And they're meant to move often!

"According to the CDC,[3] only 23 percent of US adults get the recommended amount of aerobic and strengthening activity per week to meet the minimum requirements."

When I interview my patients, I would estimate that less than 40 percent tell me that they exercise on a regular basis.

After thirty years in practice, my first line of defense, no matter what I'm treating, has been and will always be stretching. This in and of itself won't meet those CDC guidelines that are based on cardiovascular and strength exercise, but it's the easiest way to get a body moving. It can be done anywhere—anytime—and requires very little if any equipment and usually feels good!

The following pages represent phases one, two, and three of the home program. Phase one is usually assigned on the very first day of treatment if time allows, and phases two and three follow over the course of weeks or months, depending on the severity of the case and how often a patient is seen. Many of these stretches may be familiar to you, as they're yoga-based and common physical therapy stretches. I suggest you start with phase one for a period of two weeks, which should take about ten-fifteen minutes daily. Then, add phase two around week

[3]CDC (2021) Exercise/Physical Activity Chapter 4

three, accounting for an additional five minutes or so. And add phase three, which should take another five minutes, around week four. By the end, you'll have a well-rounded stretching program and a variety of exercises to choose from. Usually, over a period of a month or so, patients find their favorites and most effective ones, and they choose those on a regular basis. Just remember, even if you have very little free time, five minutes is better than nothing and can make a major difference. Consistency is the key. A little effort really does go a long way.

According to statistics compiled by goodbody.com,[4] "People often begin with yoga to improve flexibility and reduce stress." These are the key reasons they're located in this manual. It's the first tenet. Improving flexibility and reducing stress are key components of improving this condition. Also, according to these same statistics, yoga was the most commonly used complementary health practice among US adults in 2017. It's the perfect complement to any pelvic-health practice. Why are these stretches so important? Most of our leg and lower-back muscles attach to or around the pelvis, including the pelvic floor muscles. These stretches are designed to release tension and muscular tightness that is most often associated with this condition. And let's face it: being flexible in the bedroom can't be a bad thing, right?

Right! So, let's get started. Here's a list of what you'll need:

- A yoga mat or carpeted surface for comfort
- A stretching strap, beach towel, or dog lead
- A pillow if desired for head and neck support

[4]Complied by Goodbody.com Yoga

For the Restorative poses you will also need:

- A blanket
- Multiple pillows for propping/support

Optional items include an eye cover, essential oils or a scented candle, and music of your choice.

Find yourself in a comfortable, quiet location, ideally free from distractions like phones, kiddos, spouses, or partners, and (most importantly) work/stress. There are three separate assignments that fall under the "restorative" category. These poses are designed to be done for a 5–15 min time frame alone and complement the down-training pillar for stress relief and ultimate relaxation.

The following pages represent my favorite stretches and are effective for a variety of reasons. And, yes, I've personally been doing them for years—decades actually. They're assigned to address painful intercourse and a variety of other conditions. I have always said that good therapist practices what they preach.

PLEASE! It's VERY IMPORTANT that you NEVER push into your pain zone. These muscles didn't get tightened overnight, and they won't lengthen overnight. I always recommend taking the stretch to the point of a gentle feeling of elongation and holding the position for 20–30 seconds, repeating 3–5 times, 3–5x week. Stretching should always feel comfortable and pleasant. If there's any pain associated with the stretch, you're either trying too hard or the stretch isn't for you. Respect your body and be a good listener. If it hurts, don't do it. The "no pain no gain" principle is one that will NOT be applied here. And, if counting causes more stress than necessary or just seems like a distraction, just take 5–10 nice long breaths for each repetition, then relax into the stretch. You should find that your muscles gradually lengthen over time. These should produce a feeling of pleasure and refreshment. All three phases have one restorative pose attached. These can be done in conjunction with the others or as an activity in and of themselves. Restorative Yoga is a unique practice that holds the position for 5–15 min with the use of props that allow for maximum comfort and relaxation. Realize that anything you do to take better care of yourself will have a positive impact on your life and well-being. As mentioned previously, if you can only carve out five minutes, start there. So, take a deep breath, grab your mat, and let's get stretching!

Phase One

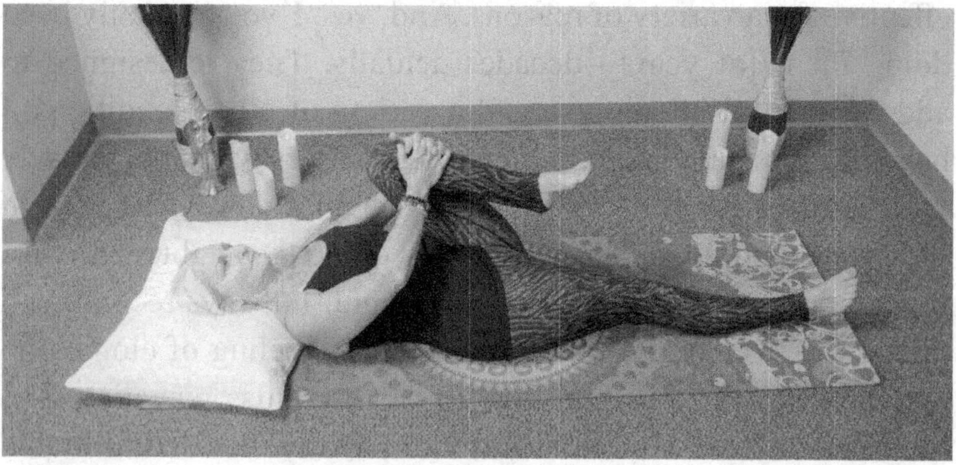

#1 Knee to chest stretch. Lie on your back with both legs extended, bend one knee and hug it into your chest. Hold for 20–30 seconds. Alternate this stretch with the hamstring stretch on the next page.

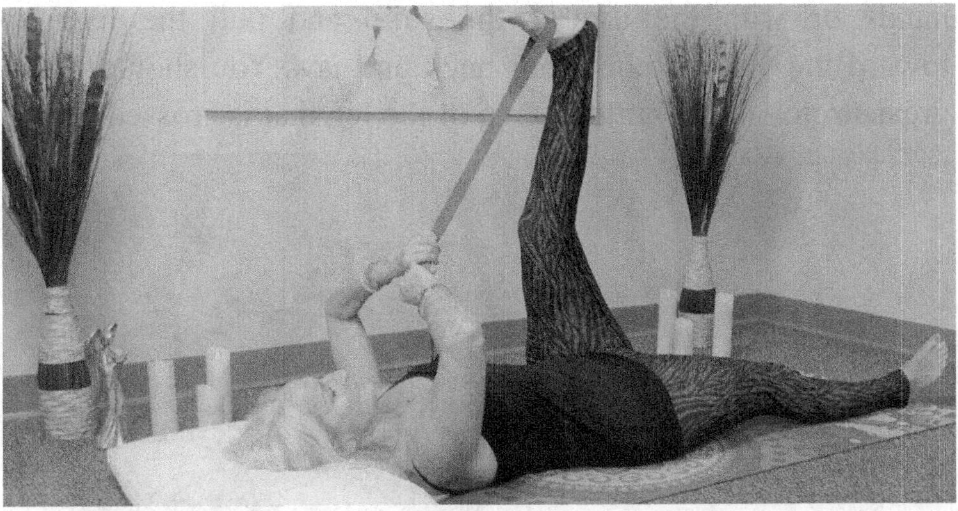

#2 Hamstring stretch. Use a strap or something similar secured around the foot and with the leg extended, but not locked, pull the leg straight up until you feel a gentle stretch along the back of the thigh. Due to the use of the strap, I suggest you alternate this stretch with the previous single knee-to-chest stretch, doing all 3–5 on one side and then changing sides.

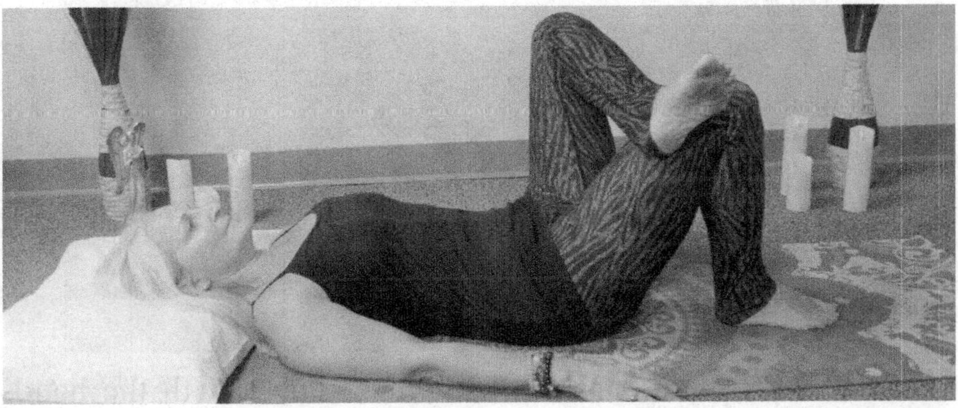

#3 Figure four. Start with both knees bent, and feet on the floor. Cross one leg over the other with the ankle resting on the thigh. Reach through the middle of the legs with either your hands or with the use of the strap and pull the legs up toward the torso. Relax your neck and jaw. You should feel a great stretch in the buttock area of the leg that is crossed.

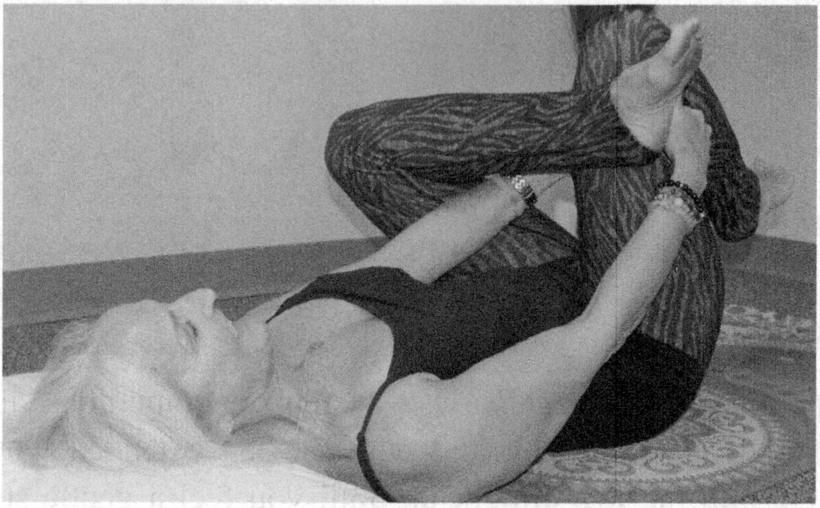

Hold 20–30 seconds 3–5x each side and then change legs.

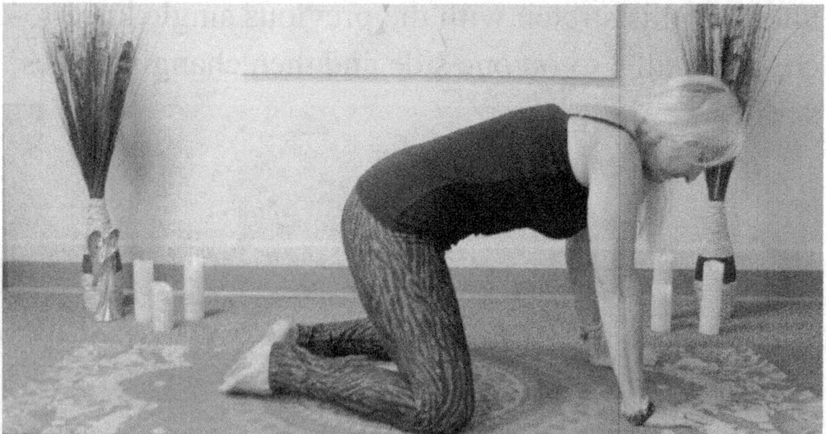

#4 Child's pose. Start on hands and knees with the hands directly under the shoulders and the knees directly under the hips. Spread the knees wide if that is comfortable.

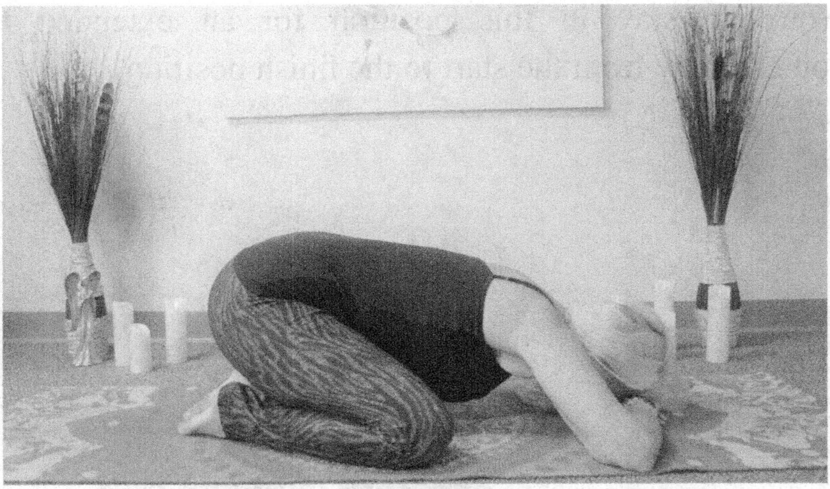

Ease your hips back to your feet and drop your head down. You may even choose to place a pillow between the hips and feet for comfort, especially if you have any knee issues. In regards to the hands, I prefer to keep my arms in the position shown above but feel free to keep the hands extended outward in front, which is more like the classic Child's pose.

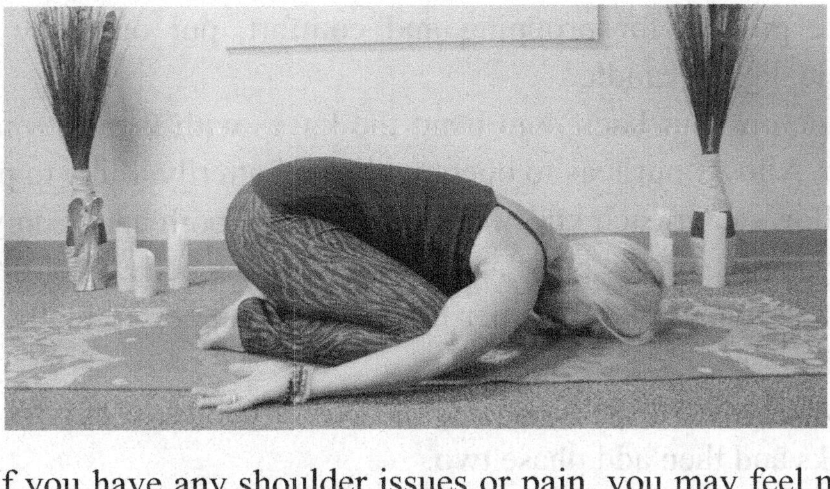

If you have any shoulder issues or pain, you may feel more comfortable with your arms extended back behind you, resting on the floor.

You can stay in this position for an extended time, or you can flow from the start to the finish position.

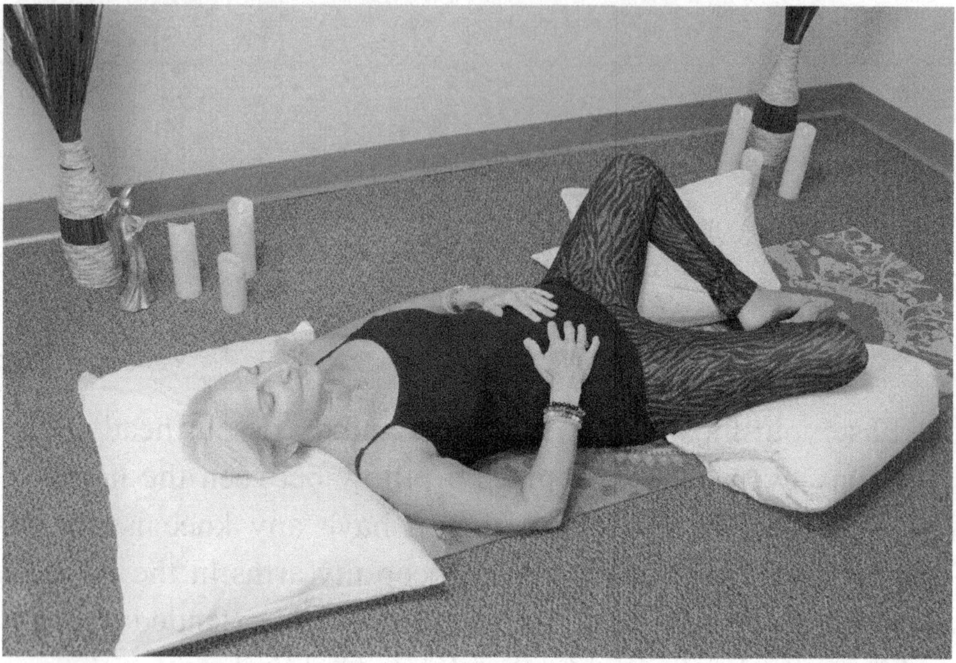

#5 Restorative pose supported butterfly stretch. Grab some pillows for propping and comfort, put on some soft music, light a candle…

Lie on your back, and bend the knees with the feet on the floor. Allow your legs to open out like a butterfly. I like to place a pillow under each knee for support. Place both hands on your belly, or one on the chest and the other on the belly. Feel free to put additional pillows under the arms for support. Breathe and relax!

Work with these basic stretches for a period of two to four weeks and then add phase two.

Phase Two

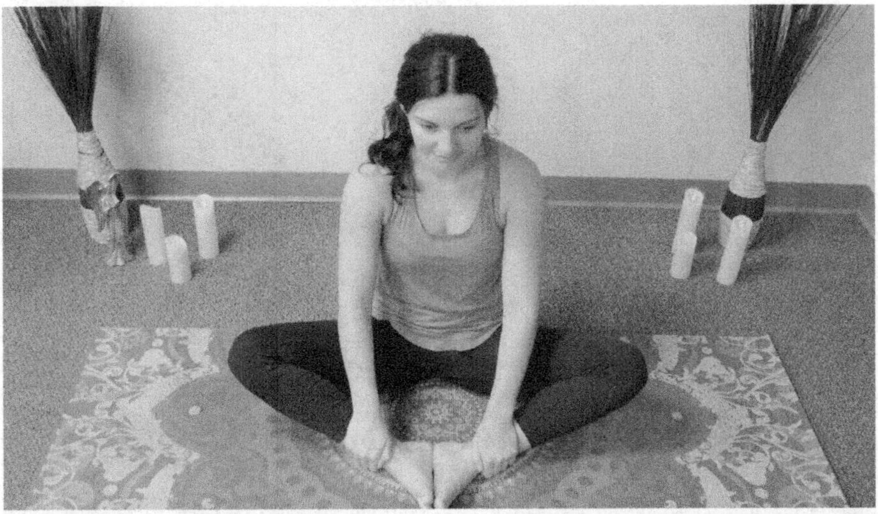

#1 Seated inner thigh stretch. Sit up nice and straight. Bring the soles of the feet together and let the knees fall out to the side. Rock side to side for 1–2 minutes.

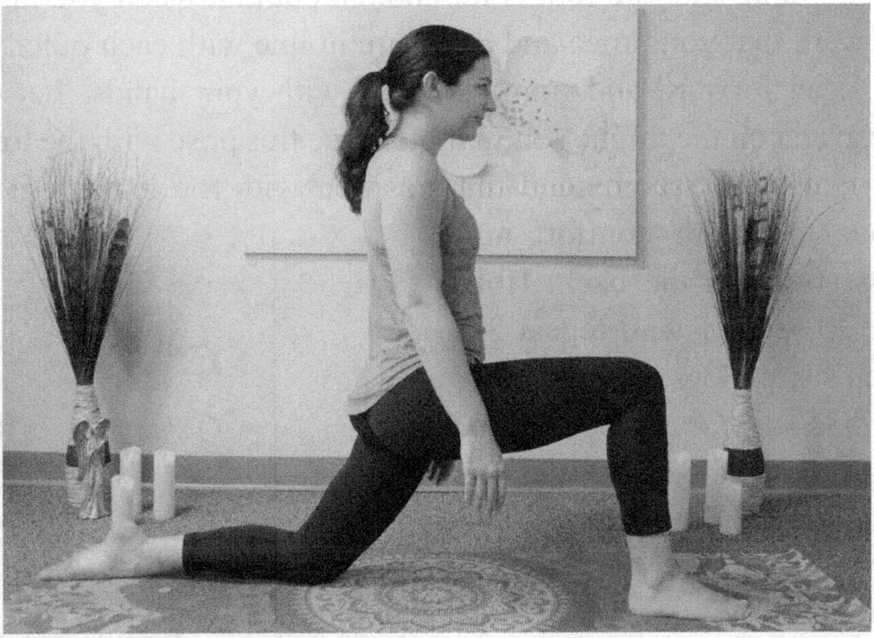

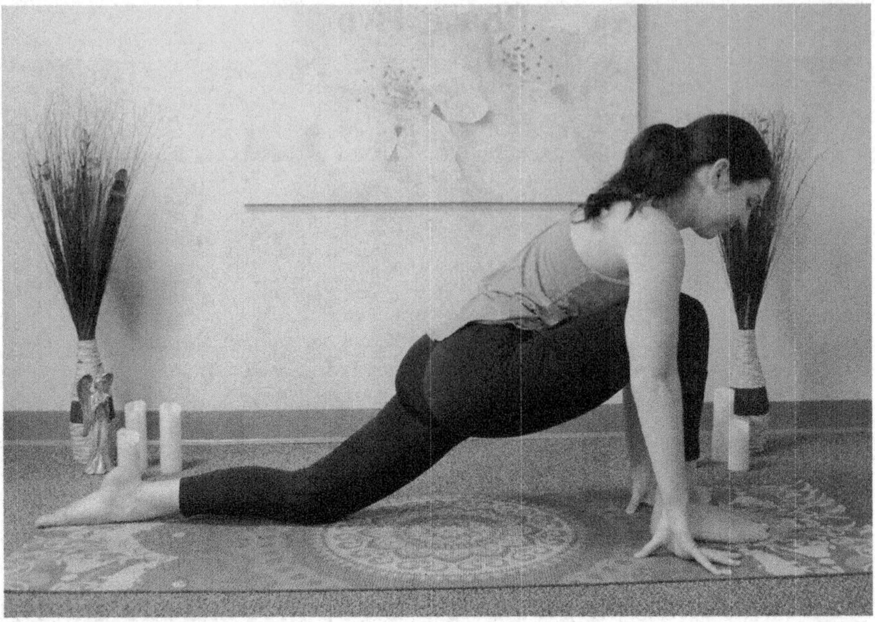

#2 Low lunge stretch. Start in a kneeling position. Bend one knee and place the foot out in front as shown on the previous page. Make sure the foot is far enough out that when you lunge forward that your knee and ankle are in line with each other.

Lean forward and frame the feet with your hands. Let the torso rest on the thigh. You will often see this pose with the torso upright but I recommend this position with the hands on the floor for more comfort and less strain on the back. Hold for 20 seconds and repeat 3x, then switch legs.

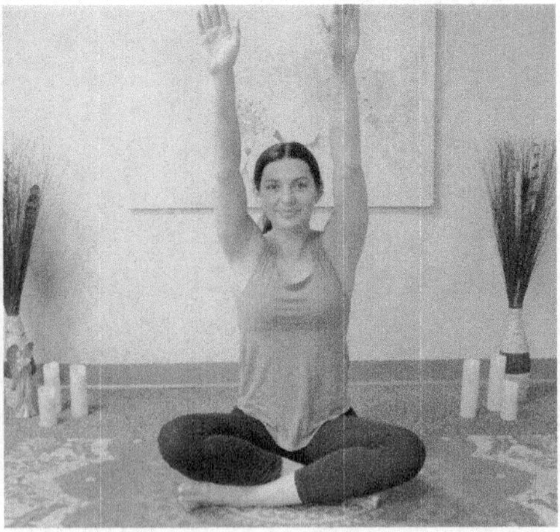

#3 Seated 3 way hip stretch. Start with the legs crossed, then take a nice breath in and reach up. On your exhale extend the arms forward.

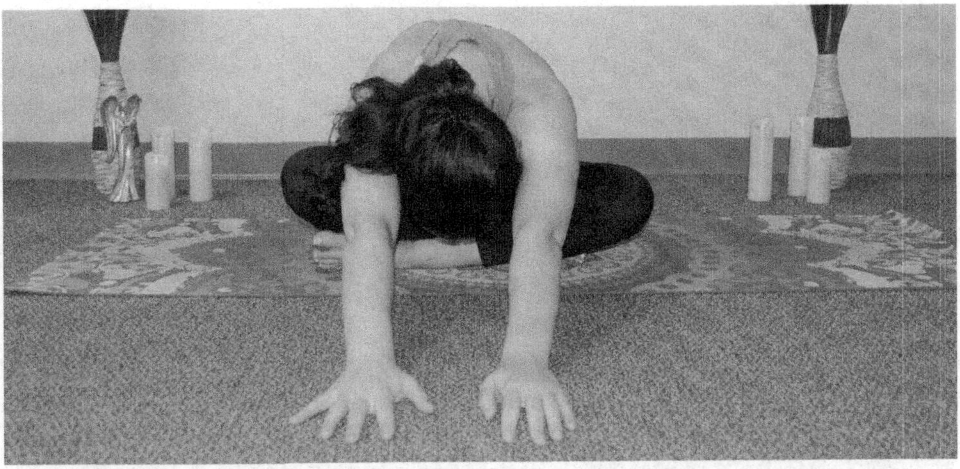

Hold for 20 seconds. Take the stretch to the right and left side.

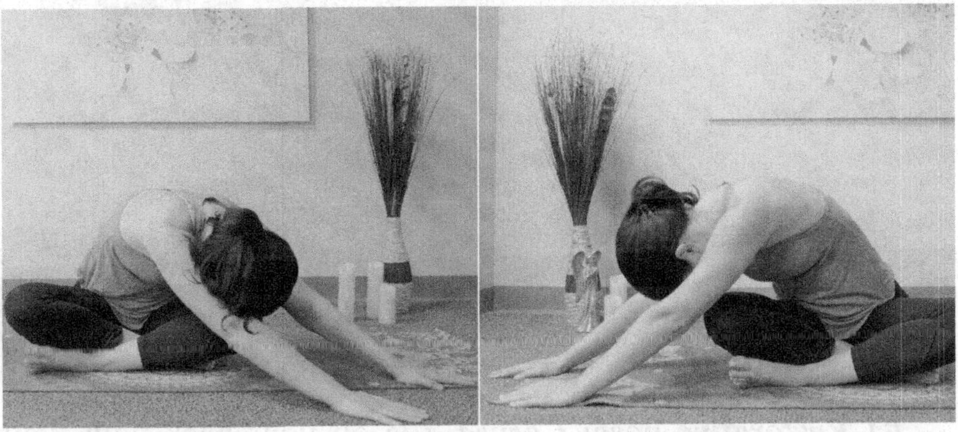

Holding for 20 seconds each, repeat 2x. Change legs, put the other leg in front, and repeat the process. You may be surprised how different the stretch feels when you change legs.

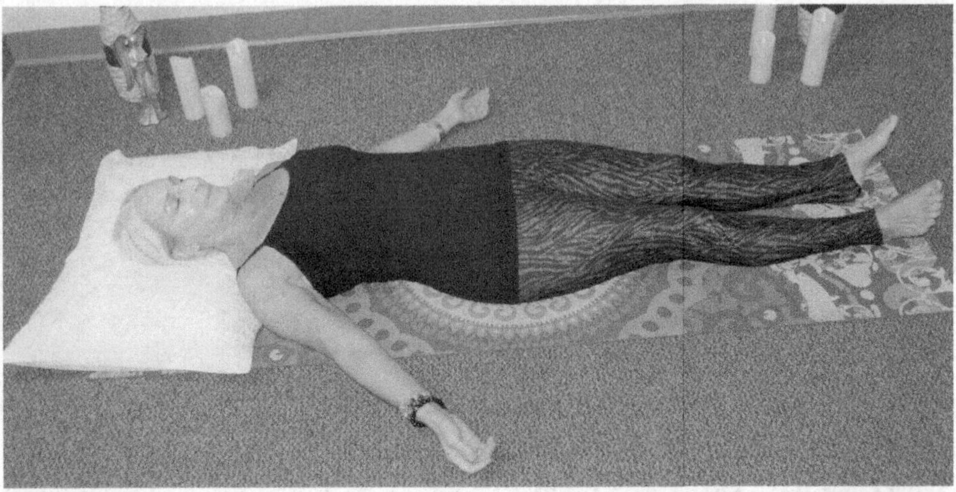

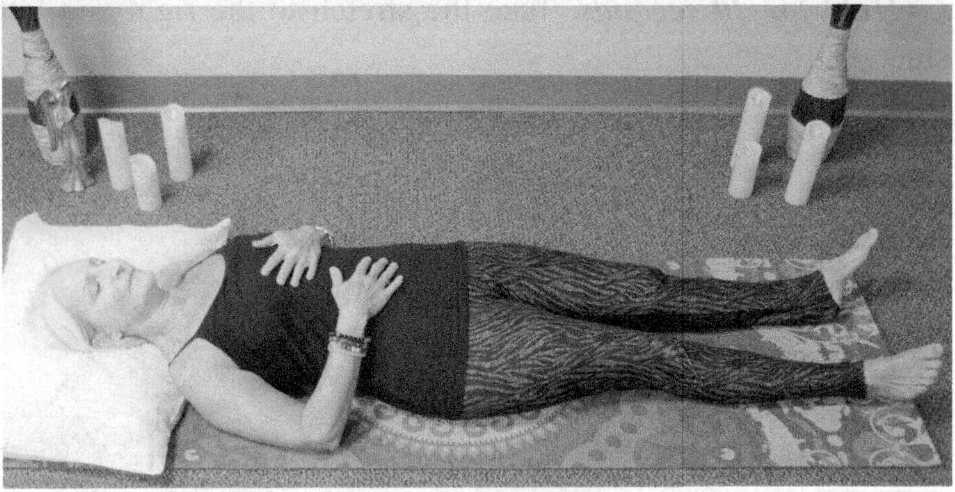

#4 Restorative pose; Corpse. Lie on your back with your arms either extended out to the side or on your abdomen. Breathe and relax!

Work with phase two for a period of two to four weeks and then add phase three.

Phase Three

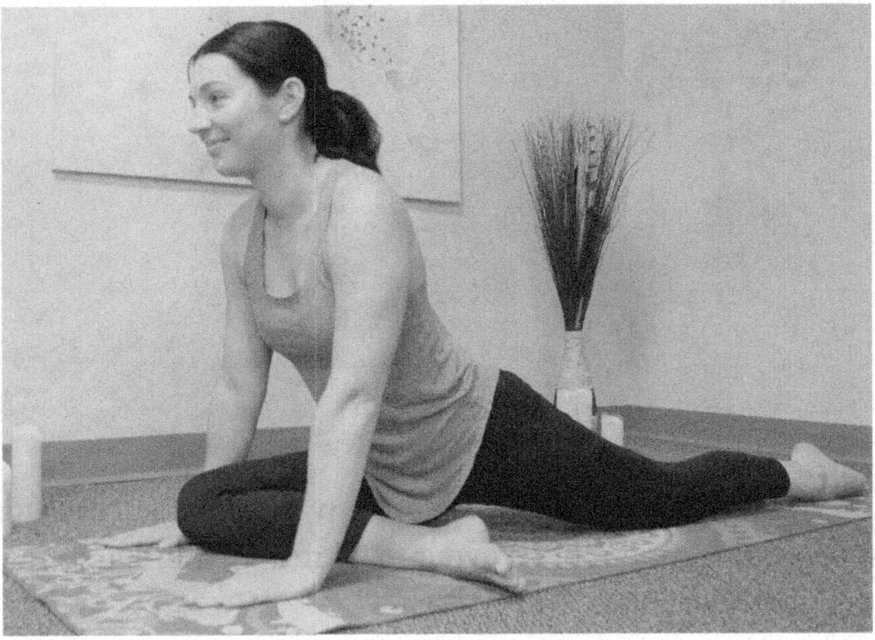

#1 Pigeon stretch. Note: this is a fairly advanced stretch. If this is uncomfortable, return to the figure four stretch in phase one.

Sit on the floor, crossed-legged. Extend one leg out behind you and keep the other leg bent at an angle that is comfortable for you. Let your hands rest on the floor support you. Relax your neck and jaw. You may stay in this position to start.

Feel free to use a block or rolled-up blanket under the hip for comfort.

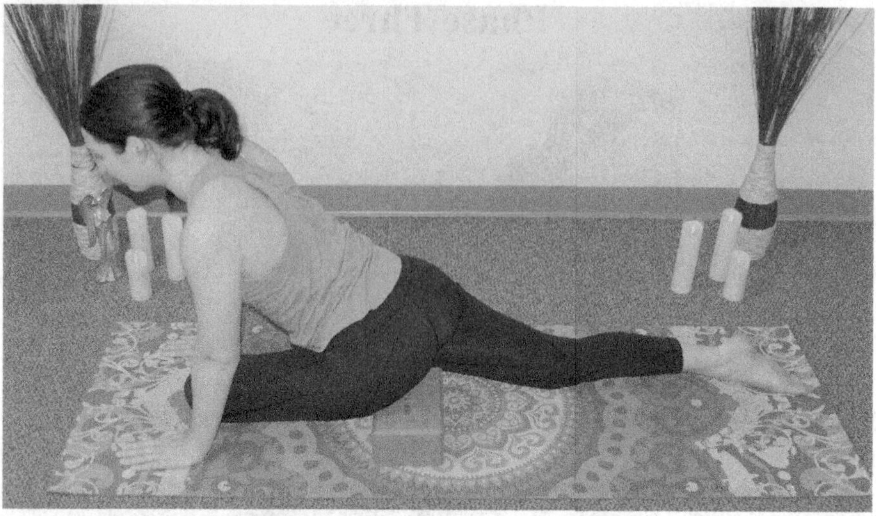

If you feel comfortable, reach out in front and let your torso rest on your front thigh. Let your head rest in your hands, close your eyes, relax and breathe.

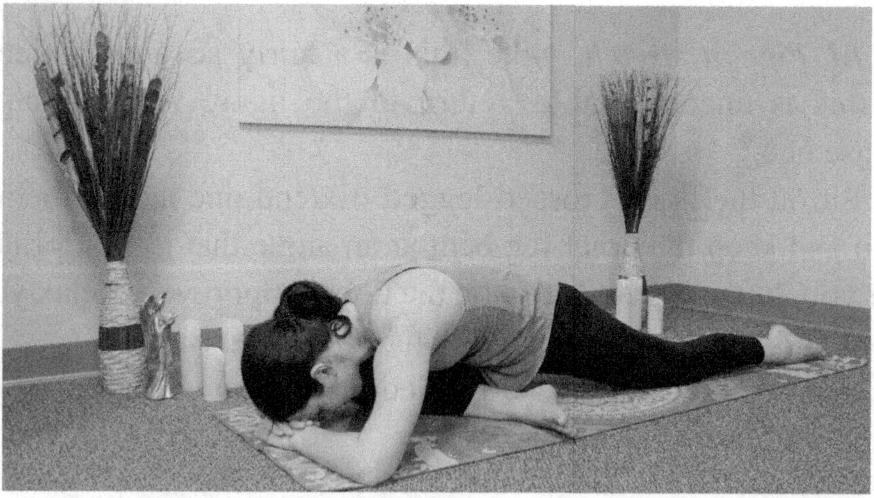

I prefer to just stay in this position for a 2–3 min period and then repeat on the other side. You are welcome to stay here longer if you like. This is a great go-to stretch when you are feeling anxious or stressed.

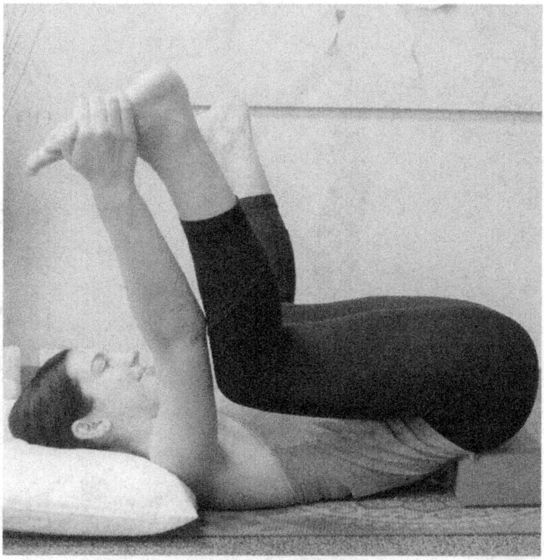

#2 Happy baby. Lie on your back and bend both knees, bringing them into your chest. Grab your feet. I like to rock side to side to get a little movement in the stretch, like the seated butterfly.

I also love using a yoga block or rolled-up blanket under the pelvis to elevate the hips. This actually allows for a deeper stretch.

IMPORTANT NOTE/WORD OF CAUTION:

If you have uncontrolled high blood pressure, a heavy menstrual flow, sciatica (leg pain), or Glaucoma DO NOT perform this exercise.

This is a wonderful pose for the ultimate in relaxation. Its benefits are many:

1. Improves circulation and swelling in the legs.
2. Relaxes the mind and body.
3. Can be helpful in the relief of leg cramps or headaches.
4. Stretches the hamstrings and low back.
5. Improves digestion.
6. Improves sleep.

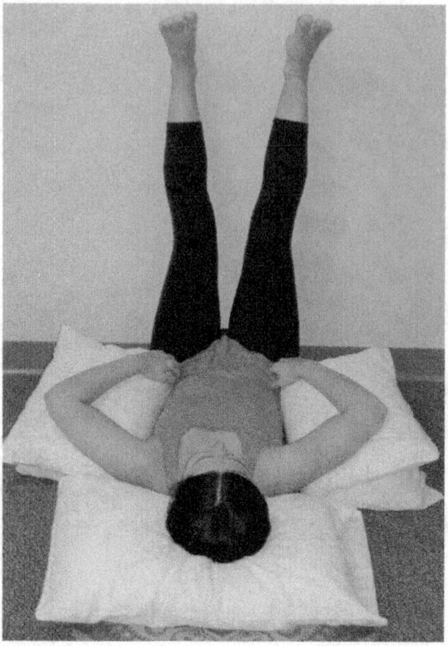

#3 Restorative pose: Legs up the wall progression. Lie on your back with support at the head and under the arms. Feel free to put a yoga block or folded blanket under your pelvis for additional comfort, you can use some eye coverings, music, essential oils, etc…

Rest the legs up on the wall. Depending on the flexibility of your hamstrings, you may be close to the wall or a bit further away. However, I do not recommend that you bring the body to a full 90 degrees, even if you can, as this can impede circulation. This pose is not designed to be a stretch on the hamstrings primarily, but simply a position of relaxation. If you are feeling a significant stretch on the back of the legs, just push out a bit away from the wall, until you are comfortable.

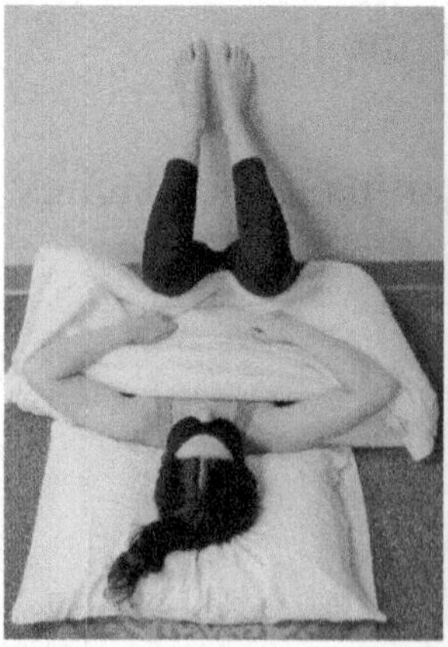

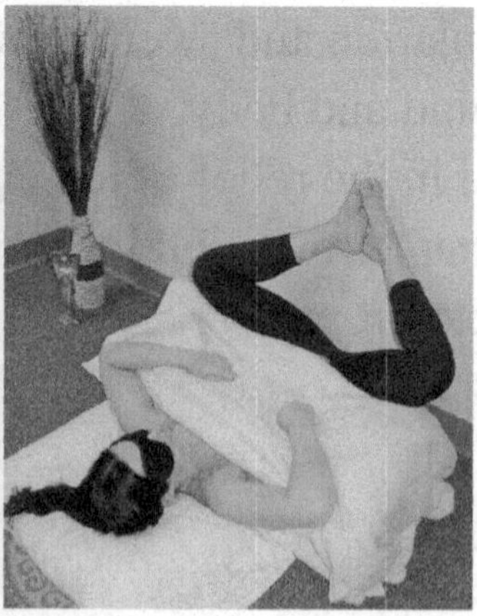

Rest in this position for 5–15 min.

Once you are ready to come out of this position, do not just get up and go on with your day. I suggest

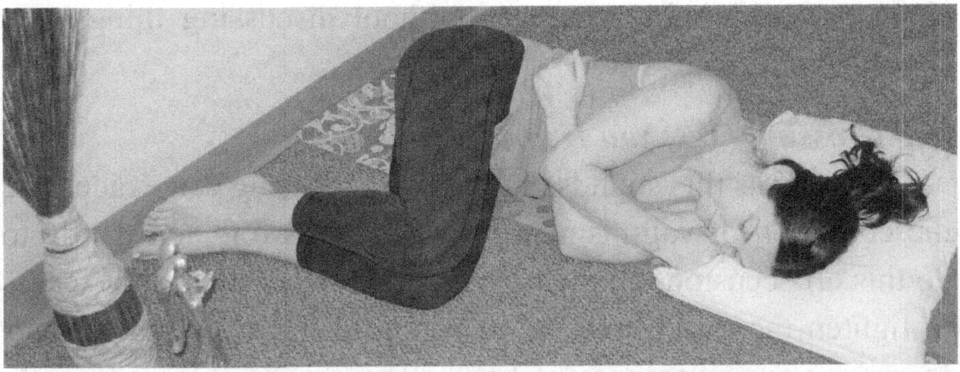

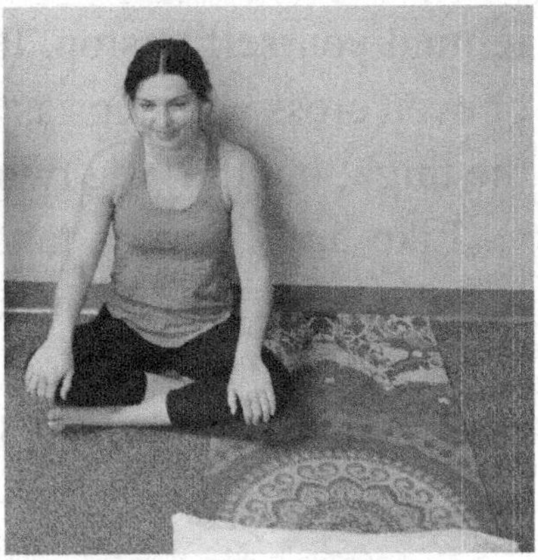

a gentle progression back to the upright posture to avoid a rapid change in blood pressure. Bend both knees and remain there for a minute or so.

You may also open the knees out to the side with the soles of the feet together for a nice inner thigh stretch.

Transition to your side and rest there for a moment.

Then transition to sitting and enjoy the relaxation response.

Smile!

See YouTube videos under painful sex no more for full-length videos on phases 1, 2 and 3.

Phase 1 ***Phase 2*** ***Phase 3***

Things to Avoid

One of the most valued aspects of seeing a physical therapist is being educated on what to do to help yourself and take an active role in the process. But the flip side of that coin is learning what not to do. This chapter wouldn't be complete without discussing things you should avoid.

Leg Crossing (Yes, You Heard Me)

As crazy as this sounds, habitual leg crossing can exacerbate the condition of vaginismus. Of course, it's fine and dandy to do this on occasion, but being a habitual leg crosser only serves to tighten the exact area we're trying to open up and release. Increase your awareness of how often you do this and gently remind yourself to stop. It's fine to cross your legs at the ankles or even cross your legs as a man might, with the ankle resting on the thigh, but the "leg twine" should be avoided.

Like any habit, it takes time to correct, so be ready for a lengthy battle. It's been said that if you do something ten times, it becomes a habit. How many times does it take not doing something to eliminate a habit? Who knows, but with patience, you've got this!

Clinching

I've found over the years that this one nugget of information can make a world of difference. Don't underestimate this information and the impact it can make! Please take notice and tune in to your body to see if this might apply to you.

Do you clench your jaw or grind your teeth? It's possible that you could be clinching your pelvic floor muscles as well. Yes, it's very common to habitually clinch your pelvic floor muscles without any awareness whatsoever. This is often a byproduct of childbirth trauma, an injury or infection, sexual abuse or assault, or hormonal changes. More often than not, though, it's associated with good old-fashioned stress—the kind of stress that makes you clench your jaw or grind your teeth ... the kind of stress that keeps you up at night ... the kind of stress that causes your central nervous system to alert the fight, flight, or freeze aspect of your brain ... the kind of stress that gives you a belly ache ... the kind of stress that high achievers and type-A personalities feel when they have high expectations of themselves and others. It can be felt in the pelvic floor (either vaginal or rectal), the glutes (buttock muscles), or the abdomen. Even holding in your stomach can tighten the pelvic floor. Remember the canister illustration? It's all a pressure system. This habit is usually something that you're not even aware of. Tenet 2 addresses this in the chapter on relaxation and down training. For now, just bring a gentle awareness to this area of your body and the possibility that you may be a habitual clincher. If you're clenching your jaw, squeezing your glutes, or sucking in your tummy, take notice of what else may be going for the ride.

Stop Doing Kegels! Seriously!

One thing I can almost guarantee is that almost everyone reading this book has heard of Kegels. Yet, the million-dollar question is this: have you ever heard of Reverse Kegels? More on this ahead! The reverse Kegels and deep breathing are key to breaking this habit and relaxing an overactive pelvic floor.

Dr. Google can sometimes do more harm than good. When you're in the market for answers, the Internet is a priceless resource and a great asset. Yet, if you've been afraid to discuss this with your doctor, friend, spouse, or partner due to the sensitive nature of this subject, be careful what you read and apply. One of the main reasons I'm writing this book is the fact that there's very little (reliable) information regarding this subject online. Yes, there's probably more out there now than ever before thanks to social media, but that being said, beware: if you're doing Kegels, stop immediately! Kegels are designed to tighten your pelvic floor muscles. It can be a practice that we apply when treating an underactive or weakened pelvic floor, but even this theory is being redefined and advanced at the time of this writing.

It's important to be able to identify the difference between a contracted pelvic floor and a relaxed one. But for the moment, let's just consider them off-limits. They do have a place in the treatment of some pelvic floor dysfunctions, but this isn't one of them. One of my patients who was in their early sixties and suffering through painful intercourse for thirty years had been doing these since her first child was born. She had no idea that this played a role in her condition. After learning and applying the principles in this manual, she was able to be with her spouse without pain after only eight weeks. At first, she didn't believe that she was going to get better. But, she's now a believer and spreading the good news to others.

Core and Strength Training (For Now)

I know this may be a hard pill to swallow, as we all want a sleek flat abdomen. But, too much of a good thing isn't a good thing at all. Heavy core exercises and/or excessive strength training like HIT often contribute to an already tightened pelvic floor area. The abdomen muscles are all attached to the pelvis and can often increase the pressure in an already highly pressurized system (again, remember the canister). Learning to relieve tension in the area of the abdomen is one of the pieces of the puzzle in addressing this condition. More on this to follow as we cover the second tenet!

The Shame Thing

Whether it was in a sex education class in middle school or the way you were raised by your good-intentioned parents, I can almost guarantee that sex and sexuality weren't subjects that were discussed often or openly. For some reason, it has always been a subject that was better left under a rock—something that most weren't brave enough to talk about. I'm not sure why so much mystery should surround something so natural. I do know that along with the shroud of the mystery lies a great deal of shame and guilt. It's the "good girl/bad girl" mindset. Somehow, we (especially women) have some deep-seated feelings about this, and it affects our relationship with the ones we love and even with ourselves.

Our society has created a deep divide in this regard. The understanding and feelings about our sexuality are multifaceted. They can be affected by where we grew up, our education, our previous experiences, our own relationship with our body, our current state of health, our present level of stress or anxiety, and our relationship with our significant other. As you can well imagine, this is dynamic and ever-changing based on numerous factors.

And, what about the notion of pleasure? It seems to be a common theme that quite often, women are not experiencing pleasure in the bedroom. As a rule, the whole notion of pleasure has been centered around men. It can be seen in pornography, in print, and in movies. The notion of pleasure has mostly been one-sided, to say the least. Well, it's time to break the cycle! It's time to embrace the sensual side of yourself and release the feelings of humiliation or embarrassment. It's time to remove the stigma and find the pleasure zone for yourself. If this is an area of apprehension, unease, doubt, or despair for you, don't feel like you're alone. There are plenty of women out there who feel the exact same way you do. I challenge you to open your mind to let go of the self-judgment. This is a time of exploration and growth. It's a time to step outside of your comfort zone and identify with a very important part of your deeper self ... your sexual self. It's time to let go of all the body judgments and explore the magic within. Connecting with your own body can serve to bring you not only closer to your loved ones but closer to yourself. Knowing what makes you feel good is at the very heart of this matter. If you don't know what feels good, how can you communicate this to someone else?

A Common Thread

Have you ever taken the Myers-Briggs (MBTI) or do you know your Enneagram number? These personality taxonomies are a great tool to help you better understand yourself and shed some light on why you feel the way you feel and think the way you think. One question worthy of serious consideration is this: Do you identify yourself as a type-A personality? As with anything in life, there is a bright side and a shadow side to everything. This is also true of a type-A personality.

On the bright side, these individuals are usually hardworking and high achievers, goal- and success-driven. They have a strong sense of ambition and are often the best leaders. They're resilient and tenacious. On the shadow side, they expect a lot of themselves and others. They're more prone to anxiety and stress. They can be impatient with themselves and those around them. They can be overly sensitive and prone to worry. They can have a hard time letting go of control and often prefer to dominate the situation.

Although not everyone that has vaginismus has a type-A personality or a penchant for perfectionism, I do see this pattern of beliefs/behaviors in my clinical practice. Some of the most common ways to address the shadow side of this personality type are to find multiple avenues for stress relief like exercise/yoga and walking, deep breathing, journal writing, music, relaxing hobbies, staying connected, and (last but not least) professional counseling from a trusted source. The principles in the next chapter are designed to calm the central nervous system and are excellent for stress management. In the meantime, take a deep breath, practice self-compassion, and stop being so hard on yourself!

Real Stories from Real Patients: LR

Would you like to tell the readers a little about yourself?

I am an active and healthy, 50+-year-old Latina. I've been married for 25 years and have 2 adult children.

How long have you been dealing with this condition and what other treatments have you tried?

In early 2020, I had to have my ovaries removed, which pushed me immediately into menopause. I didn't feel any significant difference in sexual function for about a year.

I experienced vaginal dryness, painful penetration, and painful sex. I tried different lubricants but they only helped temporarily. If we engaged in longer intercourse, I would begin to feel dry again. I would have to apply more lubricant or if the discomfort was really bad, we'd have to stop altogether.

Did you have a positive outcome/were you pleased with the results and why?

Yes! And Yes! I started to feel different. We still used lubricant but I felt that if we engaged in longer intercourse, I didn't need to reapply lubricant. It also felt like my sensitivity was increasing. As I started to feel more and more like the pain was decreasing or disappearing, we engaged in intercourse without lubricant and were pleased to notice that the pain with penetration was also gone!

Did you find the material/assignments easy to understand?

Yes. I was given handouts describing exercises that were easy to understand. We also discussed podcasts, websites, and products that could be helpful to understand what I was going through (and basically confirming that I'm not alone) and could enhance my therapy experience.

Did you find the assignments easy to implement? Why or why not?

Yes.

The exercises were simple and didn't take long.

I work from home and don't have small children so I had plenty of privacy.

I was also financially able to purchase products that would be helpful.

What were your biggest challenges and why?

Once we worked on loosening the pelvic muscles, I experienced issues with being unable to hold back flatulence. It was very embarrassing. I told Sandi about it and she changed my exercises to strengthen the pelvic floor. We had to find the right balance between loosening and strengthening the muscles.

What did you find was the easiest thing to do and why?

Exercises that I could do while I was doing something else, for example, reverse Kegels.

Would you recommend this treatment plan to others?

Absolutely! This treatment plan was life-changing for me. It has enhanced my sex life, boosted my self-confidence, and generally improved my health. I have less stress incontinence, which was an added bonus!

How long did it take to start seeing results?

About 3 weeks after I started the treatment plan.

Would you like to add anything to help the readers better understand the process and what it takes to be successful?

Be patient, it doesn't happen overnight but it will happen.

Be open. I had very open conversations with Sandi and shared extremely intimate details about myself and my sex life. This helped us develop the best treatment plan for me.

Don't keep this treatment a secret! I was so excited about this treatment and the amazing results that I spoke with my girlfriends about it. I found out one had already gone through this type of treatment and another was in need of the treatment. This is too good to keep to yourself!

5

What's in Your Head?

It's often said that a woman's biggest sex organ is her brain! Having this understanding is key when it comes to intimacy. I'd like to introduce the concept of the biopsychosocial model. This is an interdisciplinary model that looks at the interconnection between biology (the body), psychology (the mind), and social/environmental factors.

Tenet 2: Stress Management and Down Training

As stated in the Annals of Family Medicine (2004), the late Dr. George Engel, an American Internist and psychiatrist best known for the formulation of this concept of the biopsychosocial model, believed that "to understand and adequately respond to patient's suffering and to give them a sense of being understood, we must attend simultaneously to all three factors."

Let's face it: we live in an up-regulated world, full of information overload, constant contact, and multitasking. True intimacy requires learning how to switch gears and let go of the to-do list. It requires a conscious decision to get out of your head and unplug. I know this sounds counterintuitive, but being responsible for everyone and everything and trying to be all things to all people is a tall order to fill. We put a lot of internal pressure on ourselves to keep it all together all the time. It's impossible, but we hold ourselves up to this standard all too often. This in itself creates a sense of stress and anxiety that puts the central nervous system on high alert.

Again, you've heard of the whole flight, fight, or freeze thing. This is the sympathetic part of our nervous system. In and of itself, this part of our system isn't a bad thing. It tells us to eat when we're hungry, to drink when we're thirsty, to rest when we're weary, and to get warm when we're cold. It's what keeps us alert, motivated, and alive. It keeps us safe, moving forward, and growing. But if we're constantly living/residing in this system, it leads to exhaustion and creates burnout. And from what I've observed over the years, women are often at the bottom of the list when it comes to self-care. During my first meeting with each new patient, I ask the question, what would you rate your stress on a zero to ten scale if zero is total chill and ten is off the charts? Ask yourself this question. What do your rate your stress? If your answer is above a five or six consistently, it may be time to reevaluate things and consider making some changes. Living in a state of dysregulation can play havoc on your central nervous system and of course, your relationship with yourself and others.

Learning how to "turn down" the sympathetic system is only one piece of the puzzle. The real game-changer is learning how to "turn up" the parasympathetic part of our central nervous system. This system is responsible for resting, digesting, feeding, and breeding. It's why we (can) feel secure and at peace. It's our true north. Maybe you've heard of the vagus nerve, also known as the wandering nerve. This is the nerve that's responsible for our parasympathetic system. It's the longest cranial nerve in the body, and learning to befriend this nerve can serve you in ways you never imagined. Keep in mind that anything we do to stimulate this part of our brain decreases the effects of stress and anxiety. Here are a few examples of ways to stimulate your vagus nerve to promote a sense of well-being and ease:

- Deep breathing
- Meditation
- Mindfulness
- Singing, humming, and chanting
- Gargling
- Cold water to the face and neck or a cold plunge/shower
- Guided imagery
- Hypnosis
- EMDR (Eye Movement Desensitization and Reprogramming)
- Somatic bodywork
- Massage
- Gentle exercises like stretching/yoga, walking
- Shake it off (dogs do it all the time)
- Tapping
- Laughing
- Being a part of something bigger than yourself
- Sunshine
- Earthing
- Arts and entertainment
- Hobbies, etc. (Most anything that makes you feel happy or at peace with yourself and the world)

If you would like to understand more about the vagus nerve, take some time and read about the polyvagal theory introduced in 1994 by Dr. Stephen Porges, PhD, an American psychiatrist and neuroscientist.

There are also two rich free resources available at:

www.rhythmofregulation.com hosted by Deb Dana who is a clinician, author, consultant, and speaker. Her book, Anchored, How to Befriend Your Nervous System Using the Polyvagal System is a great deep dive into this subject matter. Learning how to self-regulate and co-regulate is an art and Deb has some practical advice that is easily understood and implemented.

And, www.drjoedispenza.com Dr. Joe is a doctor of Chiropractic and is an expert in mind-body medicine and brain/heart coherence. He is a researcher, lecturer, author and corporate consultant. He offers retreats, online courses and resources that cover an array of topics, all designed to help you connect to your highest potential.

So, let's talk about pain and what happens next:

Whenever we feel pain or even anticipate pain, our body responds with the production of adrenaline and cortisol. These are stress hormones and you guessed it, they stimulate that sympathetic nervous system to fight, flight, or freeze. This often creates a very shallow breathing pattern or worse yet, breath-holding. Anticipating pain with penetration immediately causes a sympathetic nervous response. Our heart rate increases, our body gets stiff, and the feelings of anxiety and fear flood in. Our muscles get inflamed. Our sex drive is suppressed. In essence, over time, you can create a hypersensitivity to this pain. Thus, learning to manage this response is one of the most important lessons you can learn in the manual.

I want to stop and take a deep breath right now.

Now, take another—slow and deep. Are you ready?

I want you to stop making attempts to have intercourse ... for now! There are many ways to be intimate with someone and share closeness and union. Be creative. You may come up with things you never dreamed of that you and/or your partner enjoy very much. This conversation can open up the lines of communication for some tender moments together to better understand the situation. The reason I'm asking you to do this is simple. Repeated attempts at intercourse that are painful aren't helping in any way. It's only feeding into the pathway from your vagina to the brain that's already overstimulated with a pain response.

Studies have shown that learning about pain and the nervous system can actually decrease your pain! Knowledge is power. You can turn your new knowledge into nerve impulses and send them to your brain. Thoughts themselves create impulses in the brain. These impulses can reframe your interpretation of the moment. It goes back to Chapter 2, where I stated that pain doesn't always mean harm. Your body is made for this and over time can respond rather than react. But for now, it's time to honor your pain. It's time to take an active role in taking care of yourself in a gentle, compassionate, and loving way. It's time to embrace your pain as a devoted mother embraces her child's pain in the most tender of ways. Recognizing that this is suffering and is no longer necessary is a very important step in healing. These exercises can transform your life and your experience of intimacy.

The following questionnaire is designed to provide you with some food for thought. It's an in-depth examination of what's in your head. Some of these questions are fairly challenging and can elicit some strong emotions. If they seem to be overwhelming, put this tool down and return to it at a later date if you desire. It isn't meant to make you feel guilty, ashamed, uneasy, or uncomfortable in any way. I've included it to allow you to look at your beliefs and feelings associated with this condition. Please consider the fact that there are NO wrong answers. As I have said to many a patient, feelings are neither right nor wrong—they just are! You're the only one to see the answers unless you choose to share them with another.

Appendix A from

Klaassen M, and Ter Kuile MM. Development and initial validation of the Vaginal Penetration Cognition Questionnaire (VPCQ) in a sample of women with vaginismus and dyspareunia. J Sex Med 2009;6: 1617–1627.

Vaginal Penetration Cognition Questionnaire (VPCQ)

Women have various thoughts and feelings about vaginal penetration. Vaginal penetration means insertion of a penis, finger (yours or your partner's), tampon and/or another object into the vagina. This questionnaire asks about your thoughts concerning vaginal penetration. The questionnaire consists of statements about vaginal penetration. You will be asked to indicate the extent to which each is applicable to you. Your thoughts about vaginal penetration are important and you can fill in this questionnaire completely regardless of whether or not penetration is possible or has ever been possible for you. There are no "good" or "bad" answers to the questions or statements. Your answer is the best when it reflects your own thoughts and feelings with regard to vaginal penetration.

Please check or circle the answer that is most applicable to you. The possible answers range from "0 = not at all applicable" to "6 = very strongly applicable."

The following is an example for clarification

Example:
I have the following thoughts about vaginal penetration:

Thought	**Not at all applicable**					**Strongly applicable**	
1. I am afraid that my vagina will not get moist (wet)	0	1	2	3	4	5	6

Suppose that you never have this thought, then you would circle "0."
You can now begin
I have the following thoughts about vaginal penetration:

Thought	**Not at all applicable**					**Strongly applicable**	
1. I am afraid that my vagina is too narrow for penetration	0	1	2	3	4	5	6
2. I am afraid that I will lose control over the situation during penetration	0	1	2	3	4	5	6
3. Penetration will feel good	0	1	2	3	4	5	6
4. Thinking about pain with penetration makes me very anxious	0	1	2	3	4	5	6
5. Penetration is a moment of intimacy with my partner	0	1	2	3	4	5	6
6. Penetration surely will not succeed	0	1	2	3	4	5	6
7. I think about everything that can go wrong and fail with penetration	0	1	2	3	4	5	6
8. I am afraid that I will panic during penetration	0	1	2	3	4	5	6

9. If I had no pain, penetration would be possible	0	1	2	3	4	5	6
10. I am afraid that penetration will become increasingly more difficult in the future	0	1	2	3	4	5	6
11. I am only a complete woman when penetration is successful	0	1	2	3	4	5	6
12. Penetration is a part of love	0	1	2	3	4	5	6
13. I am afraid that the penetration pain will get worse in the future	0	1	2	3	4	5	6
14. I feel "dirty" with penetration	0	1	2	3	4	5	6
15. I am a poor partner when penetration fails	0	1	2	3	4	5	6
16. Penetration surely won't succeed	0	1	2	3	4	5	6
17. I am afraid that the inside of my vagina will be damaged by penetration	0	1	2	3	4	5	6
18. I will become sexually aroused with penetration	0	1	2	3	4	5	6
19. Penetration gives me an unpleasant feeling in my vagina	0	1	2	3	4	5	6
20. I will be able to have a sex life that includes penetration in the future	0	1	2	3	4	5	6
21. Feeling my vagina with my own finger is scary	0	1	2	3	4	5	6
22. My partner's penis is too big for my vagina	0	1	2	3	4	5	6
23. I can easily let go of any unpleasant thoughts about penetration	0	1	2	3	4	5	6
24. Penetration will be pleasurable	0	1	2	3	4	5	6
25. I am afraid that what goes into my vagina possibly cannot come out	0	1	2	3	4	5	6
26. I am the only one in the world for whom penetration is unsuccessful	0	1	2	3	4	5	6
27. During penetration I experience a sense of control	0	1	2	3	4	5	6
28. My vagina is abnormally shaped	0	1	2	3	4	5	6

29. I am afraid of cramping up during penetration	0	1	2	3	4	5	6
30. I feel guilty when penetration is not possible	0	1	2	3	4	5	6
31. I can control the pain with penetration	0	1	2	3	4	5	6
32. The pain with penetration is caused by an illness, infection or inflammation	0	1	2	3	4	5	6
33. Penetration will result in an orgasm	0	1	2	3	4	5	6
34. I am afraid that when penetration is not successful, my partner will leave/ I will never have a partner	0	1	2	3	4	5	6
35. My mind says "yes", but my body says "no" to penetration	0	1	2	3	4	5	6
36. I am afraid that I can have no influence on what happens during penetration	0	1	2	3	4	5	6
37. Penetration will not be painful for me	0	1	2	3	4	5	6
38. It feels frightening not knowing what happens in my body during penetration	0	1	2	3	4	5	6
39. I have concerns about penetration that I cannot get off my mind	0	1	2	3	4	5	6
40. Even if penetration is not successful, I am still a good sexual partner	0	1	2	3	4	5	6

This tool can be used as a benchmark prior to applying the principles in this book and used again, after you have applied the principles. You might be amazed at the difference in your answers.

Just Breathe

Deep breathing is the easiest way to calm down the flame in the brain called pain or anxiety. It's our superpower, capable of making the quickest and longest-lasting changes in our nervous system. It's free, and it can be done anywhere by anyone for any length of time.

Check out this amazing one-minute YouTube video to see what really happens when we breathe.

Jessica Wolf Art of Breathing Demo

If you like apps, there are plenty to choose from that will guide you through the process of simple breathing/meditation:

Here are just a few to consider:

- Calm
- iBreathe
- The Breathing App
- Breathing Zone
- Headspace (for mindfulness and meditation)

Most people are fairly unaware of their breathing patterns. Generally, there are two types of breathing patterns:

Diaphragmatic (Abdominal Breathing)

This pattern occurs naturally when we're sleeping or in a relaxed state. It's slow, steady, and full. The air fills the lungs naturally and upon exhalation, exits with little or no effort. According to the American Institute of Stress, 20–30 minutes of diaphragmatic breathing can reduce stress and anxiety. According to the National Center of Complementary and Integrative Health, 12.7 percent of Americans have used deep breathing exercises for health purposes. It's usually my first recommendation to patients to help them find a deep sense of relaxation, which is essential for intimacy. I recommend that if this is fairly new to you, begin with five minutes as a starting point. I have found in my clinical practice that many patients are quite unfamiliar with breathing from the belly. If this happens to you, be patient and relax. You may even find it helpful to place a weighted object on the abdominal area to bring gentle awareness into this practice a 2 lb ankle weight, bag of rice or a stack of 4–5 magazines works well.

Thoracic (Chest Breathing)

This pattern of breathing comes from the upper chest and shoulders. It's often shorter and shallower. This often causes an imbalance in the oxygen and carbon dioxide levels in the blood, resulting in increased heart rate, blood pressure, and muscle tension. It signals to the brain a stress response, you know, the flight or fight, freeze thing again.

Diaphragmatic Breathing

Find a quiet place, free from interruption. No phone, kiddos, friends, or family. Put on some soft music if you like. You can either lie on the floor or bed or sit in a comfortable position in a chair or on the floor. Give yourself whatever support you need physically to allow your body to relax fully.

Close your eyes. Place one hand on your belly below your rib cage and the other on your chest. Allow your belly to relax and soften. Slowly breathe in through your nose, allowing your belly to gently rise and the chest to expand, then exhale through your mouth. Focus on your breath and bring your attention to the present moment.

If your mind drifts off to the past or present, gently bring yourself back to the here and now. Just let go and relax. Feel free to bring in a positive word or phrase that you repeat silently as you inhale or exhale. You even may find it helpful to inhale to a count of four and exhale to a count of four. It's even suggested that you exhale twice as long as you inhale, but experiment with the number/ratio and see what works best for your nervous system. This act of deep breathing signals the parasympathetic nervous system, which is what we want. Something to keep in mind is that the respiratory diaphragm and the pelvic floor muscles mirror one another. Having full excursion of the diaphragm will aid in getting full excursion of these pelvic floor muscles. The bottom line is that each of us responds differently to deep breathing. Please note that if you're experiencing stress or anxiety with this exercise, you may be trying too hard or putting too much pressure on yourself to "do it right." Take a break and come back when you're feeling more relaxed and try again. Never force yourself to do anything that brings you a sense of expectation when it comes to deep breathing.

Mindful Breathing

Hindus and yogis have long understood the power of respiration. In fact, while most people associate yoga with the physical poses done in a class or asana practice, the earliest texts of yoga speak to the power of the breath. Pranayama is the foundation of yoga. Prana means "life force," and yama means "control." Thich Nhat Hanh, Buddhist monk, peace activist, prolific author, poet, and teacher, describes breath as the "bridge which connects life to consciousness."

"Feelings come and go like clouds in a windy sky. Conscious breathing is my anchor. This practice involves two things: paying attention to your in-breath and your out-breath. When you breathe in, know that you're breathing in. When you breathe out, know that you're breathing out. Become aware of these two aspects of your breath—and nothing else. Make this the focus of your mind. Slowly the body and mind become one. We find oneness of body and mind in our breath."

Over time, this practice can provide us with a deep sense of awareness and freedom, allowing us to be fully alive and present—truly present. This makes us available to our loved ones and more importantly ourselves. It makes us available to encounter life in the present moment. Take this time, to really be fully present in THIS MOMENT. Running to the future or getting lost in the past, you miss life. Being present in the moment is showing up for your appointment with life. Happiness, peace, and joy are all available to us in the present moment. This door is wide open to you, waiting for you to open it. And what's on the other side may surprise you.

So, close your eyes and bring yourself to the present moment. Become aware of your body. Become aware of your breathing. Do a quick body scan. Take inventory of any stress you may be holding in your forehead, between your brows, in your jaw, your shoulders, your abdomen, your hips and pelvis, your thighs, glutes, and feet.

Breathe in and say to yourself, "I'm breathing in." Follow it all the way through.

Breathe out and say to yourself, "I'm breathing out." Follow it all the way through.

Repeat. Repeat. Repeat. Start with 5 min and build up to 15–20 minutes.

The art of mindfulness can expand to other aspects of your life as well. Try some mindful walking, mindful eating, and mindful conversation with your loved ones. It can become an art of living that brings us to the present moment.

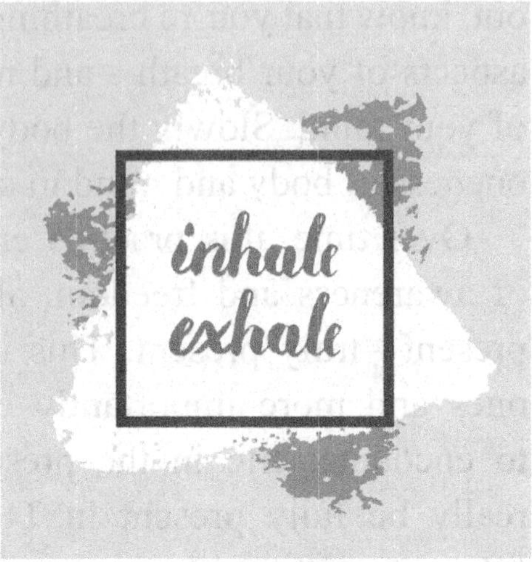

Box Breathing/Four-Square Breathing

Box breathing is often used to reduce stress and anxiety and improve mood. It's even been employed by the United States Navy SEALs to relieve stress. Known as tactile breathing, this technique can assist soldiers in dealing with high-stress situations.

Step 1 – Inhale slowly through your nose while mentally counting to four. Concentrate on filling your lungs, chest, and abdomen with air.
Step 2 – Hold for a count of four.
Step 3 – Exhale through either your nose or your mouth for a count of four.
Step 4 – Hold for a count of four.
Repeat for four-six cycles.

Again, if using the count of four feels like too much of a challenge, play with the numbers and find what works best for you. Remember, breathing should always come with a sense of relaxation. The only "rule" is that you feel comfortable with the practice.

Up for a Challenge?

Wim Hoff, also known as the Iceman, is a Dutch native who has made his name as an extreme athlete and now holds numerous world records. He's a motivational speaker and author of the book The Wim Hoff Method, released in 2020. It's comprised of three components of breathing exercises, cold exposure therapy, and mindset training. This method may not be for you, but for those up for the challenge and willing to give it a try, the benefits are manifold:

- Stress reduction
- Faster recovery from physical exertion
- Better sleep
- Improved sports performance
- Enhanced creativity
- Heightened focus and mental clarity

This method is very specific, and I recommend that you visit his website for full instructions to ensure your safety and understanding: www.wimhoffmethod.com.

What's the Best Way to Relax the Pelvic Floor Muscles?

The Power of the Reverse Kegel (Pelvic Floor Drop) and Pelvic Floor Massage.

As mentioned previously, if you've done any research about pelvic floor dysfunction, I can imagine that you have come across the recommendation to do those oh-so-familiar Kegel exercises. These are exercises that are designed to strengthen your pelvic floor muscles. Well, I can guarantee you another thing: if you do these, your condition WILL GET WORSE. This is the last thing a tight pelvic floor needs. It's important to have the ability to fully contract the pelvic floor and fully relax the pelvic floor. Having access to both extremes is key to function. But, oftentimes, the pelvic floor is so tight and shortened that when you try to voluntarily contract these muscles, you may not be able to. This is called active insufficiency. The muscles have so much increased tension that they're actually weak. This is one reason that some patients that have increased tension in the pelvic floor and experience pain with penetration may also have stress incontinence (loss of urine when sneezing, coughing, laughing, or exercising).

Under these circumstances, it's necessary to restore these muscles to what is considered a "normal resting length" before introducing any form of strengthening.

So, the goal of the pelvic floor massage and the reverse Kegel is to restore normal resting length and decrease the tension in the pelvic floor muscles. Every patient that is seen for Vaginismus is taught this exercise early on. It's key to the relaxation of these shortened, taut muscles.

How to Massage the Pelvic Floor

Beyond stretching and breathing exercises, this is usually my third assignment to aid in the down-training process. The value of pelvic floor massage cannot be underestimated.

You may choose to sit up tall in a firm chair or sit on the floor crossed-legged. I usually start with a simple hand towel that is folded in half lengthways, rolled up, and secured by 3 strips of scotch tape. This makes a roll approximately eight inches long and 3–4 inches tall, depending on the thickness of the towel. Place this under the pelvic floor area, lengthwise to cover the area from the vagina to the rectum. Shift your body forward and back and side to side to explore any areas of tenderness. If this does not elicit anything other than a feeling of pressure, I recommend that you try a football that is deflated approximately 30–40%. And yes, I know it sounds a little unorthodox but believe it or not, this surface is a perfect massage tool for this oh-so-special area. Believe me, I've experimented with numerous options to find the best choice and this one tops them all. This should be done on a carpet or a soft yoga mat. Performing this on a tile or cement floor applies too much pressure and can be quite painful. Even using a folded towel as a cushion on top of the football can be helpful if the pressure feels like it's too much. Again, just like the towel placement described above, place the ball vertically to cover the area from the vagina to the rectum. You can slowly rock forward and back and side to side—or you can make some small circles to allow the ball to massage your pelvic floor. Another option is to just sit there, relax, and breathe without movement. If you find this suggestion too painful, I suggest you return to the towel option first and then try this again at a later date. On a scale of zero to ten, the pain shouldn't be any higher than a four. Taking the time for this practice, along with some nice deep breathing is a great way to allow tension to slowly release from the pelvic floor. This activity can be done in an of itself, prior to using the vaginal trainers or prior to intercourse. The recommended time for this assignment is 5 minutes 3x a week.

See YouTube video for pelvic floor massage

How to Do Reverse Kegels/Pelvic Floor Drops

In order to relax a muscle, it can be helpful to first contract it. Here's your opportunity to do a Kegel or two. It's often suggested that you pretend you are stopping the flow of urine midstream or holding back the passing gas. It's fine to imagine that you are doing this, but actually stopping urine mid-flow is a bad idea. In order to empty the bladder, our pelvic floor

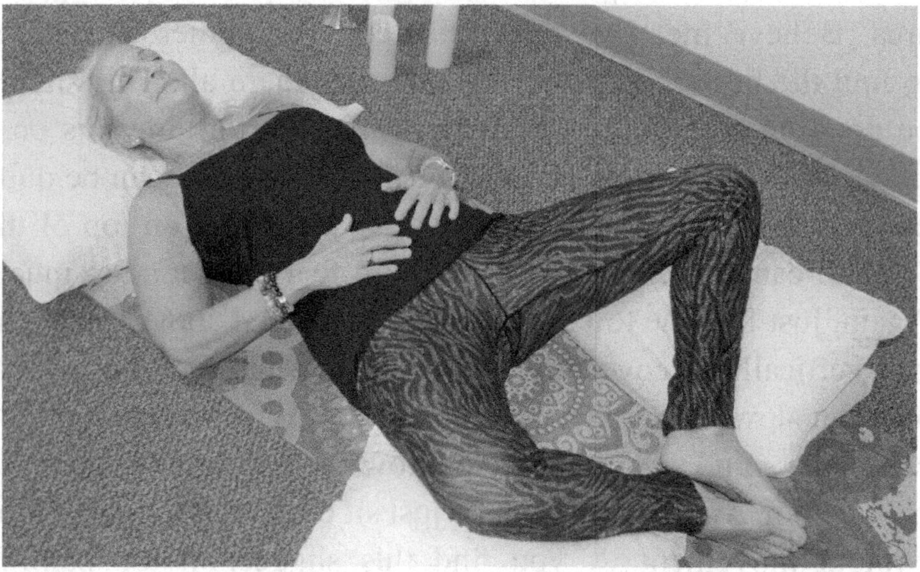

actually has to relax. For the purpose of this lesson, let's practice contracting our pelvic floor. Go ahead and try it now. Can you feel a lifting of the area around the vagina and rectum? If not grab a mirror and take a peek. You should see a drawing in and lifting up of this area. Sitting on that rolled-up towel to practice these can also be helpful. It provides some pressure in the perineal area and can be helpful for feedback to the brain.

Now, let's practice lengthening this set of muscles with reverse Kegels.

Find a comfortable supported position free from distraction. I usually suggest that a patient lie on their back, bend the knees with the feet close together on the floor or bed and allow the knees to open out into a butterfly position, like the photo seen above. Have two pillows, folded in half handy to place under each knee for support. Without the pillows, the inner thigh muscles can eventually feel too much of a stretch and actually start working against the whole relaxation process by tightening up, thus defeating the process.

Place your one hand on your lower belly, around the belly button, and the other hand on your chest. Or place both hands on your lower belly. Take some nice long deep breaths for that oh-so-familiar relaxation response. Wait for it! If you like, add some soft music, your favorite essential oils, or a candle. Let go of your thoughts, and be present in the moment.

With your next INHALATION, gently open your pelvic floor. This is done by a very gentle relaxation of the pelvic floor muscles like you are starting the flow of urine. It's a soft drop of the pelvic floor. This is meant to lengthen, release, and broaden the area of the pelvic floor. Hold for 2–4 seconds. Visualization helps. Think about the area from your vagina to your rectum. All of this area needs to go along for the ride, not just the vagina. For your reference, if you go back to the picture of the pelvic floor on page 10 you'll see that anatomically, the larger muscles of the pelvic floor are actually in the area around the rectum. You can imagine the pelvic floor like a bowl or balloon that's slowly, softly opening, or expanding outward. You can visualize the area between your sitting bones softly spreading. You can focus on the area between your pubic bone/tailbone expanding and opening up. DON'T PUSH DOWN. Some therapists even like to use the analogy of an elevator. At rest, we are on the ground floor. Contracted, we may rise to the first or second floor. A reverse kegel is descending to the basement. It's extremely important that you don't strain yourself. This effort is very minimal and relaxed. Repeat this exercise for 2–3 minutes two times per day. This is also your go-to exercise to address clinching. Whenever you notice clinching or tension in this area, do a few reverse kegels to help release undue pressure.

Tips

- Always do this exercise with an empty bladder and bowels.

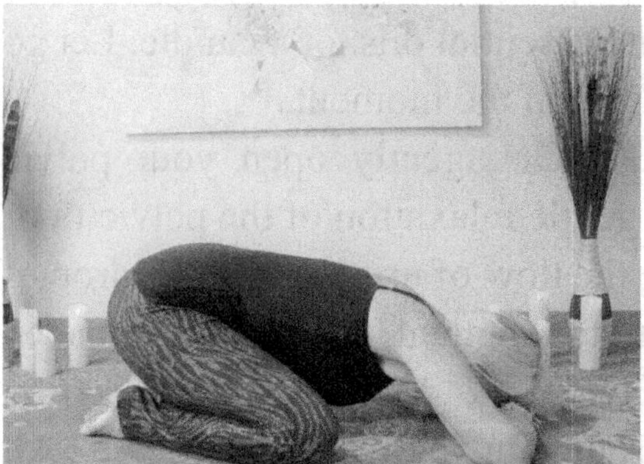

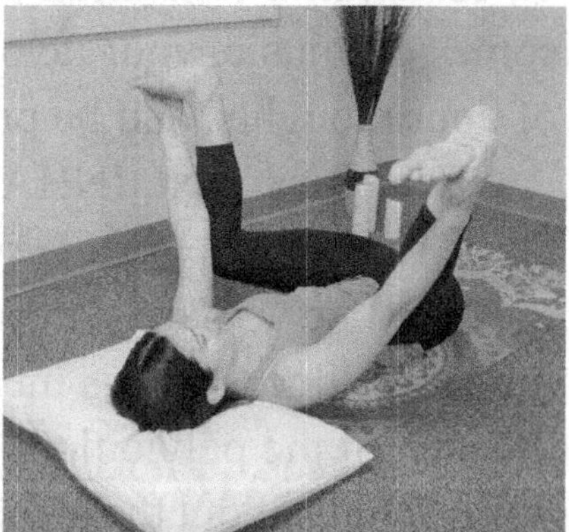

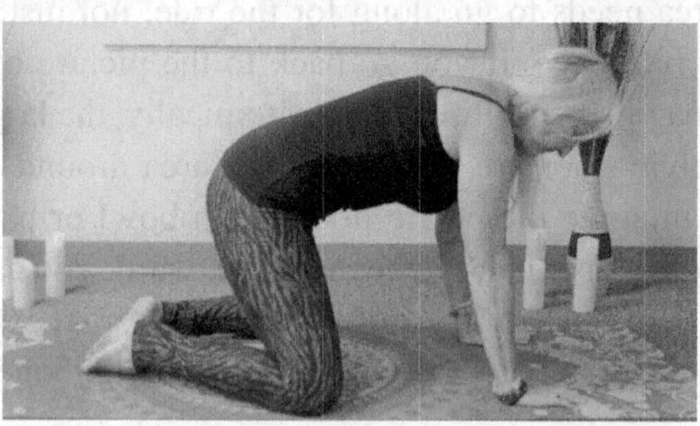

- Consider using a mirror for feedback and to better visualize the process. With the reverse Kegel, you should see the area between the vagina and rectum (the perineal body) move downward toward the mirror.
- Remaining shallow, place your finger into the vaginal opening to feel the gentle expansion of the pelvic floor as you inhale and release.
- Alternate positions: try this process in Child's Pose and or Happy Baby; consider on hands and knees or in a supported squat position. Each of these positions offers a different feeling, and some are assisted by gravity. Find what works best for you.
- Once you've mastered this, check in with your pelvic floor throughout the day for any tension or clinching. Use this technique to relax those muscles during a busy day or during times of increased stress.
- These can be a great addition to foreplay and should definitely come prior to penetration.
- There are a great number of videos that can further assist you in learning this extremely important exercise. One that I'm quite fond of is led by Denise Conway at www.theflowerempowered.com. Denise is an insightful, knowledgeable yoga instructor and personal trainer that seems to have a love for the pelvic floor and sharing her own personal story about her pelvic floor dysfunction. Her mission is to break the taboo surrounding pelvic floor dysfunction. She also has some great videos on YouTube that you might find handy in conjunction with the next chapter, which centers on self-care strategies.

In 2021, she released a book and an eight-phase training program, Empower Your Flower. Although this addresses all pelvic floor dysfunctions, other than pelvic floor tightness, she does devote an entire section to this particular condition. Look for content regarding lengthening or relaxing the pelvic floor, not strengthening or prolapsing.

Pelvic Floor/Abdominal Relaxation Using a Yoga Block or Blanket

You'll need a yoga block. I prefer the three-inch variety. If you don't have a yoga block, grab a folded-up blanket or pillows that will lift your hips up off the floor approximately three inches. Lie on the floor with your knees bent hip distance apart and feet on the floor. Lift your hips into a bridge. Place the yoga block/blanket/pillow under your sacrum. This is the area between your lower back and your tailbone. Place the block/blanket in such a way as to allow your pelvic bones to be in what is referred to as a posterior tilt. Think of a bowl of soup that you want to drink out of that's tilting toward you or having your tail tucked. It's important that your back not be arched and this should remain pain-free. If it's painful, this probably isn't the best option for you, and you should move on to other options.

If you do find this comfortable, allow your pelvis to be supported by the prop. Just sink into it and feel the gentle suspension of all your pelvic organs and your pelvic floor. Breathe and relax. This is actually a perfect position to do some gentle abdominal massage. This in itself can provide some much-needed release of any tension that may be being held in this region. I like to take both hands and begin at the level of the heart. Take your hands and apply gentle pressure, following the outline of the bottom of the rib cage on each side. Make a sweeping motion outwards towards the bottom of the ribs, around the waistline. Repeat a few times and then work your way down to the belly button and then all the way down to the pelvis/pubic bone. This can be done with alternating hands, right and then left, or in unison. Repeat until you reach the pelvis, then work your way back up. If you find any one area of increased tension or tenderness, spend a little more time there and give this area some loving attention.

After 2–5 minutes, lift your legs up, grab your knees, and gently open your legs out into a wide V. You can provide support with your hands by allowing your elbows to rest on the floor and hold your outer thighs or just keep holding onto your knees.

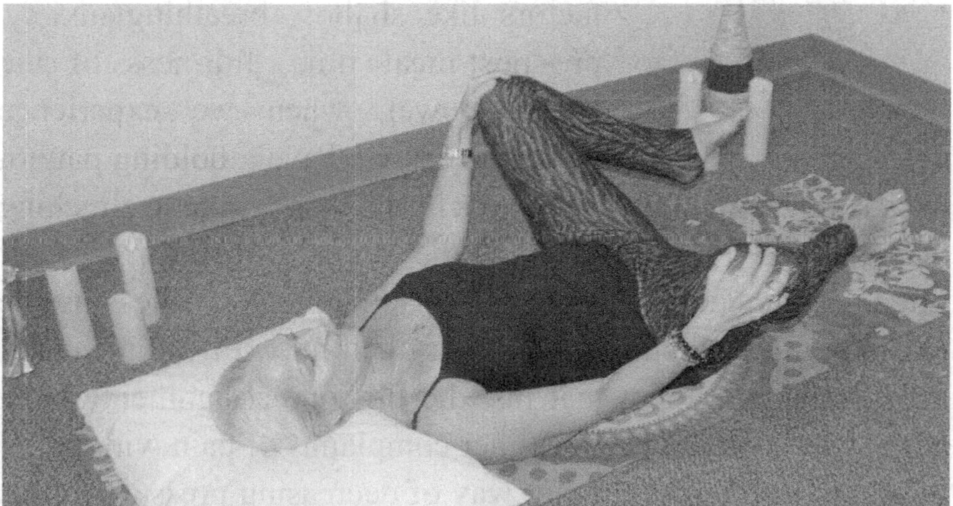

You can also provide some gentle pressure on each inner knee to increase the intensity of the stretch. Making large circles with your legs in this position can be quite comfortable and relaxing as well. I personally love this whole sequence and the relaxation response it produces. Perform 5–10 circles in each direction. If opening up the legs seems a bit too much, just return to your starting position with feet on the floor and let this be your personal option.

Everybody Loves a Good Belly Rub!

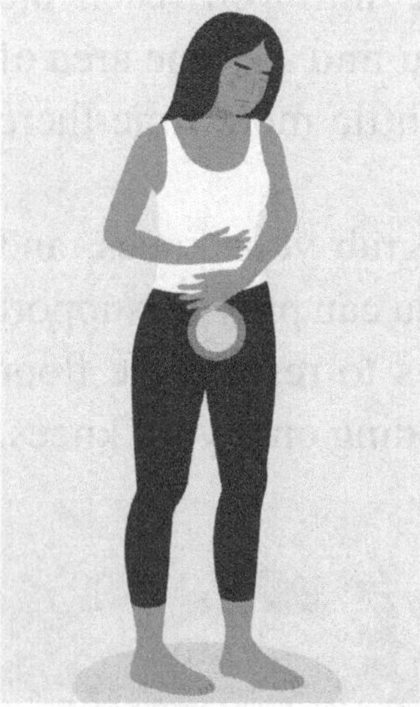

If you consider the area from your diaphragm to your pelvic floor, remember, it's all under pressure—sometimes too much pressure!

At any one time, we have around twenty-two pounds of pressure in our abdomen. It's just the nature of our system. This varies based on a number of factors like shallow breathing/anxiety, pre-/post-meal time, full-ness of the bladder/bowel, when we experience pain or when we have a holding pattern of "sucking it in". This "sucking it in" habit is similar to clinching of the pelvic floor muscles and they often go hand in hand. It often goes unnoticed—like many bad habits. Yet, releasing the tension in the abdomen can be very helpful with vaginismus. I actually had a patient that just did this one assignment alone, and it was enough to address her complaints of pain with initial penetration. It's just another way of decreasing pressure in this already highly pressurized system. My favorite choice is to take a small nine-inch soft Pilates ball that isn't fully inflated. The cost of this is $10 or less. It's very important that this ball be very soft to adapt to the softness of the abdomen. If you're able to, lie on your stomach, propped up on your elbows, and in line with your shoulders. Place the ball under your abdomen. Start just below the rib cage and just move your body back and forth, allowing the ball to massage the diaphragm, located just under the rib cage. After a few minutes, take the ball and move it very slowly right down the middle of the abdomen from the center of the rib cage to the belly button, all the way down to the pubic bone. If you find any tender spots along the way, stop and breathe into it. Stay long enough to allow the tension to release. Move downward until you reach the pubic area. There is actually a structure from the belly button to the pubic bone; it's called the urachus and can often hold a lot of tension. Pay close attention to this area. This may all be a new feeling that you have never experienced, but give your body some time to adjust, and it can be quite effective. Try 3–5 min, and remember that a little goes a long way. Some patients even find that this aids in elimination and promotes bowel movements.

See YouTube video for abdominal release

The Role of Constipation

Although not a pleasant topic of conversation, constipation isn't an uncommon complaint among patients that are treated for vaginismus. As previously noted, the larger muscles of the pelvic floor are located in the rectal triangle, which is found from the bottom of the vagina to the rectum. Increased tension in these muscles not only makes intercourse difficult but can also play a role in the ability to pass stool. Often, patients applying these principles will notice an improvement in their complaints of constipation, not realizing the connection. If you truly suffer from constipation, make sure to mention this to your therapist. Here are a few simple suggestions that can make a world of difference:

- Consider getting a Squatty Potty, which is designed to make bowel movements easier.
- Staying hydrated is key. Try to drink at least 6–8 glasses of water per day.
- Try and consume twenty-five grams (for women) and thirty-eight grams (for men) of fiber per day. Food sources like vegetables, fruits, and grains are your best options, but you can use fiber supplements sold in a variety of forms: powders, gummies, and pills. I suggest that you gradually add any of these into your system. It is possible that it may bulk up your stool making it harder to pass. Pay attention to how you respond and realize that everybody is different. A supplement may not be for you.
- Consider using a stool softener. These are a type of emollient and can often be just enough to do the trick. The number-one pharmacist recommendation is Colace. You can start with one and add an additional dose (up to four per day). This can be used short-term for the purpose of avoiding straining the pelvic floor during a bowel movement. Chronic straining of the pelvic floor can lead to organ prolapse, and managing constipation is your first line of defense in protection from this.
- Experiment with different positions: lean forward, lean back, lean to the side ... everyone's sigmoid colon (the end of the tube) is shaped differently. Not ideal for a

long term management is MiraLAX and Smooth Move/ Senna tea. Also something to consider is magnesium citrate, but check with you pharmacist or health care provider if you are taking other supplements; this is not to be used if you are on a SSRI antidepressants.

A side note: I also use the abdominal massage techniques for patients that suffer from constipation. Using this technique daily can aid in elimination. If you're using it for this, use the pattern below.

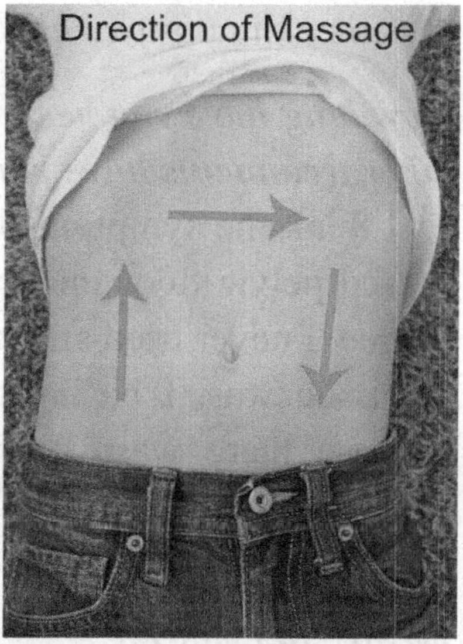

Move from the right lower abdomen, up and across under the ribs to the left side of the abdomen. This pattern follows how our digestive system works: from the ascending colon to the transverse colon to the descending colon to the sigmoid colon to the rectum.

Or just lie on your back in a comfortable supported position and use a tennis ball, hand-held massage tool, or your own fingers to explore this area. If you find tender spots or areas of increased tension, apply just enough pressure to be meaningful and therapeutic. Apply pressure for a minimum of 90 seconds to allow the area to melt and soften. And as always, BREATHE! Our goal is to release tension and promote a softness in the area of the entire abdomen.

Real Stories from Real Patients: MR

Would you like to tell the readers a little about yourself?

I am a woman in my early 30s, originally from the Midwest but have moved around the country chasing career opportunities. I went to school for Aerospace Engineering for both my undergraduate and graduate degrees and I am currently working in the space industry at my dream job. I am married to a wonderful and caring husband, who is also an engineer, and we are both currently working hybridly between our offices and at home with our two cats.

How long have you been dealing with this condition and what other treatments have you tried?

I think the symptoms began about five to six years before I started pelvic floor therapy when I was pursuing my Master's degree. I never tried any treatments because I didn't know what the issue was. I hesitated to bring it up to my gynecologist because there wasn't consistent pain, and I never had any abnormal OB-GYN visits, so it just didn't seem that serious.

Did you have a positive outcome/were you pleased with the results and why?

Before going to pelvic floor therapy I was almost completely unaware of what the pelvic floor was or what could be causing my issues. I had a very positive outcome! I learned about the pelvic floor, and we discovered the root cause of my symptoms, and sex was no longer painful for me. I also now have the tools and knowledge to work back to remain symptom-free.

Did you find the material/assignments easy to understand?

The materials and assignments were easy to understand. I was given stretches to do to loosen up the muscles connected to the pelvic floor.

Did you find the assignments easy to implement? Why or why not?

Yes and no. The stretches were great but did take quite some time if I went through all of them, so it required some self-discipline to work them into my daily routine.

What were your biggest challenges and why?

My symptoms started because of stress, which will continue to be a challenge for me because stress is so unavoidable, and it will take time for me to work on controlling my body's automatic responses to stress.

What did you find was the easiest thing to do and why?

The easiest thing was actually going to the appointments every week. I was very comfortable chatting with Sandi, and I could tell she knew what she was doing and she was working out the painful area of my pelvic floor.

Would you recommend this treatment plan to others?

100%.

How long did it take to start seeing results?

I think it took at least 6 sessions to start feeling the symptoms lessen, and 9 or 10 for the symptoms to be gone.

Would you like to add anything to help the readers better understand the process and what it takes to be successful?

The first appointment with the therapist was more of a get-to-know, which was good because we ended up spending a lot of fairly intimate time together. We talked about my symptoms and when they started occurring. I was also given the option whether to have an initial exam to find the location(s) causing me pain. It was eye-opening to feel the different muscles almost individually, especially after seeing the diagrams of the pelvic floor for the first time.

After my painful area was pin-pointed, I had weekly pelvic floor massages that would aim to essentially massage the painful area, kind of like a typical massage removing muscle knots. And during those massages, we would talk a lot, it almost acted as a therapy session for me too. Together we figured out the root cause of my pain, which was the stress I had put on myself both academically and at work throughout the years. The stress caused me to clench my pelvic floor muscles without me ever realizing I was doing it. Compounding that tension over the years led to the pain in the pelvic floor, which was only noticeable during intercourse. In hindsight, it makes a lot of sense, and now I do recognize and feel my pelvic floor tensing up when I'm stressed.

I was given a list of stretches to do to loosen my hip and groin muscles between visits to the physical therapist because, as I learned during my sessions, all of those muscles are connected to the pelvic floor. The stretching also helped quiet my mind a bit as well, which helped counteract the stress. The stretches did take some time to work through, and I was never really into yoga or other forms of stretching, so I had to work them into my daily routine to make sure I did them regularly.

It took about two months of physical therapy and stretching at home to undo the tension in my pelvic floor muscles. Before I started physical therapy I felt awful turning away my partner's advances because I just wanted to avoid the pain of having sex. With the stress of the COVID-19 pandemic making sex more and more painful for me, I finally decided enough was enough and I wanted a solution to my problem. I'm glad I had an understanding gynecologist that pointed me to pelvic floor therapy and am extremely grateful that I had a caring, kind, and knowledgeable pelvic floor therapist that I could trust. She helped me figure out the cause of my issues and gave me the tools and knowledge I needed to no longer have painful sex.

6

Self-Care Strategies

Tenet 3: Self-Care Strategies

This chapter is by far the most important in this manual. It provides the fundamentals of how to address this condition. The previous chapters are meant to educate and provide a framework from which to begin. This chapter is all about self-care. And let's face it: mental health is definitely getting some much-needed attention, kind of like the pelvic floor ... finally. And self-care is a hot topic of conversation in mental health circles. It's about taking care of yourself mentally, physically, emotionally, socially, and spiritually. It's another aspect of the biopsychosocial model spoken of in the previous chapter.

Self-care has been defined as "a multidimensional, multi-faceted process of purposeful engagement in strategies that promote healthy functioning and enhanced well-being."[5] And of course, I think we can all agree that if we're not taking

---

[5]Dorociak KE, Rupert PA, Bryant FB, Zahniser E
Development of Self-Care Assessment for Psychologists.
Journal of Counseling Psychology 2107; 64 (3) 325-334

care of ourselves, we can't be our best selves—i.e., our true selves. I recommend that you begin any of these techniques after you've taken the time to perform some of the down-training principles presented to you in the previous chapters. It's extremely important that you're as relaxed as you can be. Being in an up-regulated/stressed state will only act as a barrier. You want your body and your mind to be in a receptive state. If nothing else, just take a few minutes to do some deep breathing and spend a few minutes massaging your abdomen.

The following tool provides an ideal opportunity to stop and take a look at multiple areas of your life that contribute to your sense of well-being: It addresses physical, mental/emotional/spiritual, professional/work, and social/family. It's an inventory of multiple levels and changes as factors in our lives change. Of course, as we grow and change, it also changes. Feel free to refer back to this tool as often as you like and see where you have made some positive changes that are making an impact on your sense of well-being and happiness.

Self-Care Questionnaire

Patient Name ______________________________ Date ____________

Research shows that people who take time to recharge and restore are more creative, happier, and more successful. This questionnaire will help you identify the areas of your life that are well-tended and those that could use more time and attention. This is not meant to be a diagnostic assessment. Instead, it is a tool to help you see what you are doing to care for yourself. There are no right or wrong answers to these questions, and some of them may require a bit of thought. Take your time and answer each question to the best of your ability based on your self-care practices right now.

Instructions

For the following questions, please rank each item on a scale of 0 to 5, as follows:

0 = never 1 = rarely 2 = sometimes 3 = often 4 = regularly 5 = always

Physical Wellbeing — How often do you:

1. ______ Eat a whole foods-based diet rich in colorful fruits and vegetables?
2. ______ Drink enough water?
3. ______ Exercise for more than 20 minutes?
4. ______ Wake feeling refreshed from sleep?
5. ______ Sleep at least 7 hours per night?
6. ______ Make time to relax or nap?
7. ______ Take time to breathe deeply throughout the day?
8. ______ Engage in stress-reducing activities (excluding TV or screen time)?
9. ______ Spend time in nature?
10. ______ Feel nourished, healthy, and strong?

Physical Wellbeing Total: ______________

Mental, Emotional, Spiritual Wellbeing — How often do you:

1. ______ Make time to participate in things you enjoy?
2. ______ Give and receive affection regularly?
3. ______ Feel understood and valued by those who are close to you?
4. ______ Feel gratitude on a daily basis?
5. ______ Find meaning in life even during difficult times?
6. ______ Take an interest in or find joy in the world around you?
7. ______ Have hope that things will get better?
8. ______ Express yourself creatively?
9. ______ Treat yourself with kindness?
10. ______ Remember to make your dreams and goals a priority?

Mental, Emotional, Spiritual Wellbeing Total: ______________

For the following questions, please rank each item on a scale of 0 to 5, as follows:
0 = never 1 = rarely 2 = sometimes 3 = often 4 = regularly 5 = always

Professional Life, Work, Career — How often do you:

1. ______ Hold a work position in an area of your interest?
2. ______ Work in a position that matches your professional goals?
3. ______ Find a sense of meaning and enjoyment in your work?
4. ______ Empathize and connect with customers, clients, and work colleagues?
5. ______ Have confidence in your ability to address challenges in your professional life?
6. ______ Feel supported at work or in your professional life?
7. ______ Have someone you can rely on if you need help or guidance?
8. ______ Set limits at work, whether it be with clients or tasks?
9. ______ Disengage and leave pressures behind at the end of the day?
10. ______ Take vacation or holiday breaks to allow for some downtime?

Professional Life, Work, Career Total: ______________

Social Life, Family, Relationships — How often do you:

1. ______ Have a dependable person who listens to you?
2. ______ Have supportive family and friends close by?
3. ______ Get enough social time with people who make you happy?
4. ______ Participate in group activities with people who share a common interest?
5. ______ Spend time with people who make you laugh?
6. ______ Feel like your close relationships are loving and supportive?
7. ______ Have the ability to say no comfortably?
8. ______ Do something fun with family or friends at least once a week?
9. ______ Feel like your personal life brings balance to your professional life?
10. ______ Feel comfortable asking for help when you need it?

Social Life, Family, Relationships Total:________________

Score Interpretation and Next Steps

The higher your score in each section, the better you may be at taking time for self-care and wellness in each aspect of your life. Trying to improve your scores can help create more balance in your life.

Consider items on which you scored 3 or lower. How can you modify your behavior to improve your self-care practices? What goals might you need to set in order to make these changes?

____

____

____

____

____

____

Based on Transforming the Pain: A Workbook on Vicarious Traumatization by Saakvitne KW, Pearlman LA, and the staff of TSI/CAAP; 1996.

Now, it's time for something very important...

So what's really driving this feeling of pain with penetration? It should be noted that pain with initial penetration is reported considerably more than pain with deep penetration, in my experience. This is due primarily to the superficial muscles of the pelvic floor. Contrary to what you might think, these muscles aren't actually in the vagina. They're the muscles surrounding the opening in what's referred to as the vaginal triangle.The vagina itself actually has no muscles. It's a canal that extends from the vulva to the neck of the uterus (cervix). The wall contains layers of elastic fibers and rugae, which are pleats of extra tissue that allow the vagina to expand during intercourse and childbirth. The superficial structures that surround the vaginal opening are the superficial/deep transverse perineal, ischiocavernosus, bulbospongiosus, and introitus (opening of the vagina). I know that's a lot of fancy jargon, but in the industry, we refer to them as the STP/DTP, IC, and BS for short.

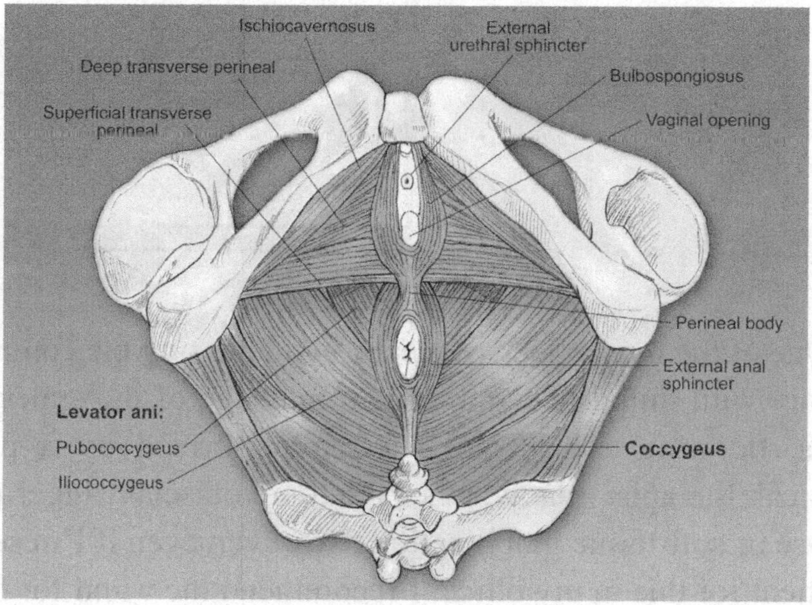

When these muscles perceive a threat and send signals to the brain, this emits pain. In turn, these muscles tighten protectively, and the rest is history. Let's change history with these self-care strategies. Keep in mind that these muscles, like any other muscles, can and do respond to stretching, relaxation techniques like deep breathing, reverse Kegels, and massage. I promise! Trust the process and keep in mind, this is not a race, it's a journey.

Introducing the Pelvic Wand

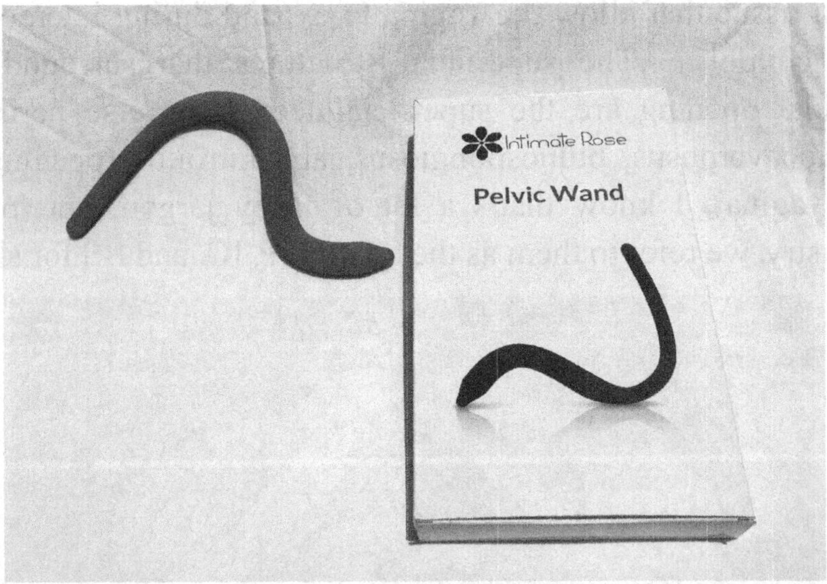

One of the most effective means of addressing the complaint of pain with initial penetration is a massage of the superficial pelvic floor muscles. This is often performed by a pelvic physical therapist via what's called myofascial/trigger-point release or soft-tissue mobilization. However, even if I'm seeing a patient for this in my office, I recommend the wand for home use as well. With or without the option of seeing a therapist, it's the best tool for the tension release of superficial pelvic floor muscles. It's important to understand that this particular set of muscles isn't deep. As noted, the muscles aren't in the canal but around the opening. The depth of these muscles is literally only ¾–1 inch.

And the reality is that it isn't about the wand; it's about YOU introducing a non-threatening stimulus that you control. It helps by providing a means to decrease tension in the muscles, which provides local and centralized desensitization. This is a key concept referred to as graded exposure. This is a process by which you slowly and progressively expose yourself to a form of stimulus, in order to make you less sensitive to that form of stimulus. It can literally change the way that the nervous system perceives the threat. The tissue learns to adapt to the demand. Beyond pain, two of the most common words used to describe what occurs with initial penetration are burning and stinging. These are nerve signs. The nerves of the pelvic floor are sensitive to pressure—often hypersensitive due to repeated attempts at painful intercourse. The wand is truly the best tool to decrease this sensitivity ... until I invent something else.

The pelvic-massage wand is my number one and first recommended accessory for addressing the superficial pelvic floor muscles and nerves. My favorite is made by Intimate Rose. This handy device is made of smooth and soft medical-grade silicone designed by Amanda Olson, DPT, PRPC, a pelvic floor therapist. I recommend the extra cost of investing in the vibrating option, which has ten different vibration choices. I will say that the vibration is fairly strong, so if you are sensitive purchase the regular or heated option. This wand also has two ends to choose from—one smaller and one larger. It might be less threatening to start with the smaller end although I find the thicker end to be the best choice.

Vibration is used for four primary reasons:

1. Vibration increases blood flow, thereby, bringing oxygen-rich blood to the area for more receptivity.
2. Vibration is used in physical therapy as an inhibitory agent. This means it decreases the tension in the muscles, making them more relaxed. (Sounds like a good idea, right?)
3. Vibration provides an alternate stimulus to the pain that has been felt in the past to help throughout the desensitization process.
4. Vibration can be used as a toy for clitoral stimulation.

Using a wand is much easier than beginning with dilators, which are inserted into the vagina for stretching the introitus (opening) and can be quite intimidating. Although this wand is designed to reach the deep-hip muscles (called the obturator internus) and the deeper pelvic floor muscles (like the puborectalis and iliococcygeus), I most often recommend that the wand be used at a depth of approximately 1 to 1 ½ inches, just near the opening of the vagina—specifically the superficial muscles that surround it. It should be mentioned that EVERY patient says the same thing. They are surprised and often in disbelief that this area is the source of the problem. They all perceive that it is deeper, inside the vagina. If you use the wand as described below, you will find that over time, these muscles will relax and lengthen, allowing for initial penetration to be comfortable.

As mentioned, if you do any search on the Internet regarding how to use these wands, you'll most likely see that it's inserted into the vagina and used on the deeper muscles mentioned. I however prefer to use it in the fashion described on the following page, to release these more superficial muscles that make initial penetration painful. I have found the wand to be VERY effective and easy to use, especially for women who have done little or no self-exploration or minimal exposure to the use of toys.

If this is your first time using any type of device around this area, I can guarantee you that it will feel foreign and a bit uncomfortable at first. Just be prepared and know that you're in a safe place, in control of the stimulus, and I promise that it gets easier with time and practice. Just give the process a chance. It works!

So, let's get started...

First of all, wash your wand with soap and warm water. Then, gently dry it. Have some water-based lubricant handy to allow for gliding over the tissue. Oil-based will degrade the silicone. Ideally, the lube should be free from parabens, sulfate, and propylene glycol. It's important to find a time when you know you will not be distracted or disturbed. It's helpful not to be in a hurry, as feeling rushed doesn't equate to relaxation.

I recommend that you lie on your back propped up by several pillows to place you at a 45-degree angle or so. The bottom line is that you don't want your abdominal muscles to be engaged, which will only serve to tighten the pelvic floor. You should be able to easily reach your hands to your vulva without activating your core muscles. Open your legs like butterfly wings (yes, I love my butterfly position). Take two additional pillows, folded in half, one for each side, to place under the knees to support. This additional support will allow for the relaxation of the adductor muscles. These are the inner thigh muscles, and the fascia (a type of connective tissue) from these muscles blends into the pelvic floor. Just like the abdominal muscles, we want these muscles to be relaxed.

To begin, spread the outer labia to expose the deeper tissue around the inner labia and vaginal opening. Use a small amount of water-based lubricant around the tip and approximately one inch down for ease of glide. Visualize the area of attention like a clock. The bottom of the vaginal opening is 6:00. My experience is that the area from 4:00 to 8:00 is the most common site of pain and tightness. This will be your primary focus.

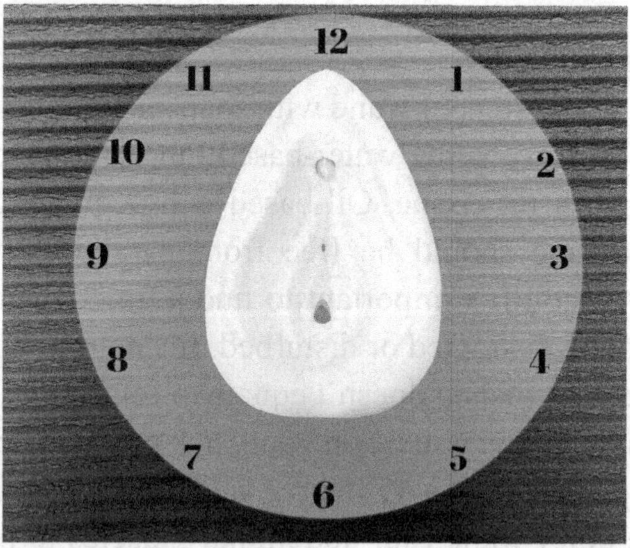

Explore each side of the clock separately and search the area for tenderness. Gently explore and press into this tissue which should release some of the tension or tightness. Don't press too hard to create a strong pain response, but make sure to press hard enough to identify the muscles that need attention to make it therapeutic. Remain in the area of concern for a minimum of 90 seconds or longer and breathe into it. The muscles that you're trying to identify are those STP/DPT, IC, and BS muscles that you learned about earlier. There's also an area of concern called the perineal body. This structure lies between the vaginal and rectal openings. It can often elicit a pain response due to the taut nature of this structure. It's very important that if you get anywhere close to the rectal opening, you remain in this area, working on the areas of tension that you may find. Don't return to the upper area around or within the vagina. This can open up the chances of cross-contamination or infection. The bacterial flora of the vagina is sensitive and should be treated as such.

As previously mentioned, these superficial muscles and surrounding tissue are the ones that make initial penetration painful or sometimes virtually impossible. Another way that this device can be helpful is to gently insert it into the vaginal entrance approximately one inch deep to find the introitus or vaginal opening. This is an excellent way to begin to stretch this tissue, allowing for easier entry. Start at the bottom at the 6:00 position. Stretch downward and hold for at least ninety seconds. Then, move around the clock. I find again that most of the increased tension can be found from 4:00 to 8:00. Feel free to explore around. Be cautious, and don't apply pressure at the 12:00 position toward the belly button. This is your urethra, which is the bottom of the bladder where urine is stored. And yes, there are three holes "down there."

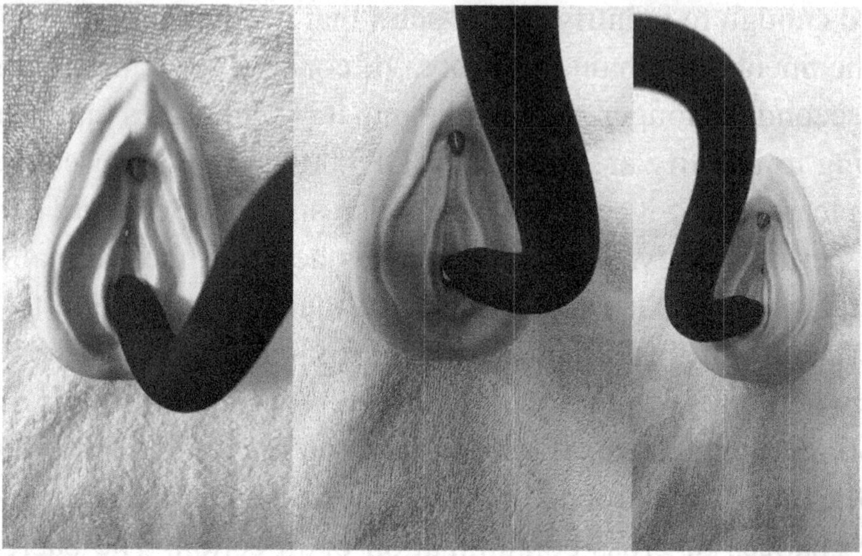

Go to www.intimaterose.com/SANDI1 for a direct link for $5 off.

See YouTube video how to use the pelvic wand

Beyond the Wand

Feel free to use a little lube and your own thumb or fingers to explore this area as well. These manual therapy techniques are what pelvic floor therapists do in the clinic, and they're truly some of the most effective means used to address the complaint of pain with either initial or deep penetration. Whether you're using the wand or your finger/thumb, take your time and be patient.

This is something I recommend doing for 5–10 min or so, 3–4 days per week. It can be an activity in and of itself, used prior to dilator use, or a pre-intercourse routine. I've even had patients use it as a part of foreplay. And remember: don't push into the pain zone. On a scale of 0–10 with zero being no pain and ten being "take me to the hospital" pain, try not to let your pain go above a three or four. If it hurts, just back off the pressure in the same location of restrictions and remain there until it relaxes. I usually recommend that a person stays at the tender point until it releases and then goes a little deeper until such time that it feels like pressure rather than pain. You can also change the angle of the wand to be more specific or effective. It may initially be a bit uncomfortable, but being slow and steady is the key to success. Take a deep breath and trust the process.

Once pain-free initial penetration is achieved, you may find that deep penetration is a concern. As mentioned previously, this wand is specifically designed to reach these deeper pelvic floor muscles. If you're a visual learner, The Intimate Rose website and the Ohnut Pelvic Gym have some excellent instructional videos that are easily accessible. Or just do a web search on how to use the pelvic wand. There are numerous other sites that provide guidance. And if you're concerned about harming your internal organs with this deeper technique, let me assure you that your bowels, bladder, and uterus are located well above this area and there should be no concern of injury.

To address the deeper structures, I recommend the same position described previously. You'll need a bit more lubricant to cover the entire end up to the curve. Gently insert the wand into the vagina to the point of the curve. Begin by using a sweeping motion, starting at the 6:00 position and sweeping toward 10:00; then, sweep from 6:00 to 2:00. If you find any tender spots, stay there until you feel the tissue respond by relaxing. It should feel like your finger sinking into a firm stick of butter, melting away into softness. You can toggle back and forth to assist in the relaxation response.

One deep hip muscle that can refer to pain with deeper penetration is the obturator internus, an internal rotator, located on each side at around the 3:00 and 9:00 positions. This muscle may come into play if you've had a hip injury or labral tear in the hip joint. The wand is an excellent self-management tool to get to this itch you feel like you otherwise can't scratch. If this muscle gets your attention, once you find it, you can also gently rotate the hip in and out, bringing the knee toward the body and out to the side. Doing this allows the muscle and the movement to do the work, rather than moving the wand.

Explore a bit and see what works best for you. A final word on pain with deep penetration: if your pain is located near the rectal area, you may have a coccyx (tailbone) misalignment or hypomobility (decreased motion) component. This condition needs the expertise of a pelvic floor specialist, ideally one that is skilled in rectal assessments and manual therapy in this area. Not all therapists offer this option, so be sure to do your homework.

I suggest using the wand for a period of 2–4 weeks prior to vaginal trainers/dilators, depending on your history.

If you want to see some additional videos on the use of the wand or dilators, check out a resource already cited: Denise Conway with www.theflowerempowered.com (also available on YouTube). She has some nice instructional videos on techniques to relax the pelvic floor. Look under the drop-down knowledge, and choose Sexual Dysfunction for some educational reading material as well. Look under the News drop-down, which will lead you to the latest content regarding vaginismus, pelvic floor relaxation, and beneficial stretches. The information on strengthening or hypopressive exercise is designed for those with prolapse or incontinence due to an under-active pelvic floor, not an overactive pelvic floor. These are not recommended for vaginismus.

Another Explanation for Pain

At times, the length of the vagina can be shorter than the length of the penis. Or the cervix may ride low or be tilted. If this is the case, your sensation will feel like your partner is hitting a wall deep down in the lower abdomen/pelvis. It can result in excruciating pain. This can also occur if there is any kind of prolapse. If this is the case and what you're experiencing, it could possibly be the cervix.

There is an amazing product on the market called, OHNUT.

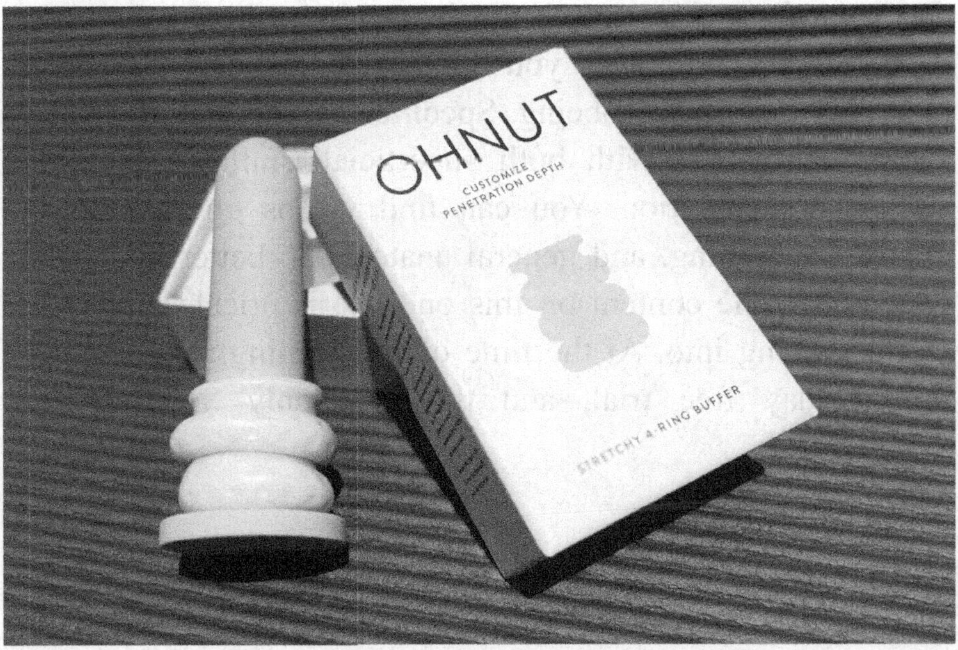

You can find them on www.ohnut.com. This handy little product is doctor-recommended and partner-approved. Emily Sauer, OHNUT Founder and CEO, came up with the idea out of necessity. She had been experiencing pain with deep penetration for years and just thought it was something she just had to deal with (like so many women do). She came up with the crazy idea of putting a pink frosted doughnut on the penis. This was the beginning of her mission. These comfy, modular soft, squishy rings incrementally adjust to create a buffer for custom depth penetration. In 2022 she added a new option, the vibrating Oh Nut. It acts as both a buffer and a cock ring for pleasure. OHNUT also offers the Pelvic Gym. This online program offers users access to twenty renowned pelvic floor physical therapists. There are fifteen motivating curated programs with 800+ minutes of content—including pelvic floor classes that are constantly being updated. There are a number of programs to choose from, but with respect to the subject at hand, you'll want to explore the content regarding Sexual Well-being. Specifically, you can find videos about painful sex with both superficial (initial) penetration and deep penetration. You can find videos on how to use dilators, stretching, and general anatomy to better understand your body. The content on this one site is priceless and well worth looking into. At the time of this writing, you can do a fourteen-day free trial, and then it's only $10/month or $90 per year.

At Last, It's Time: Dilators/Vaginal Trainers

Let's face it: A vagina should be able to accommodate a tampon, a finger, a sex toy, a speculum for an internal exam, menstrual cups or discs, and if desired, a penis. The pelvic floor muscles should be mobile and flexible, just like any other muscle.

And although the thought of penetration can certainly cause fear and anxiety, the use of a vaginal trainer is the best way to introduce penetration in a safe, controlled fashion.

Remember, the goal of all this is to desensitize this area in such a way to provide stimulation that you control.

Let's cover some frequently asked questions:

What are vaginal trainers?

Vaginal trainers are cylindrical in shape and vary in size by length, circumference, and diameter. They're usually available in 6–8 graduated sizes, each getting larger in all three measures.

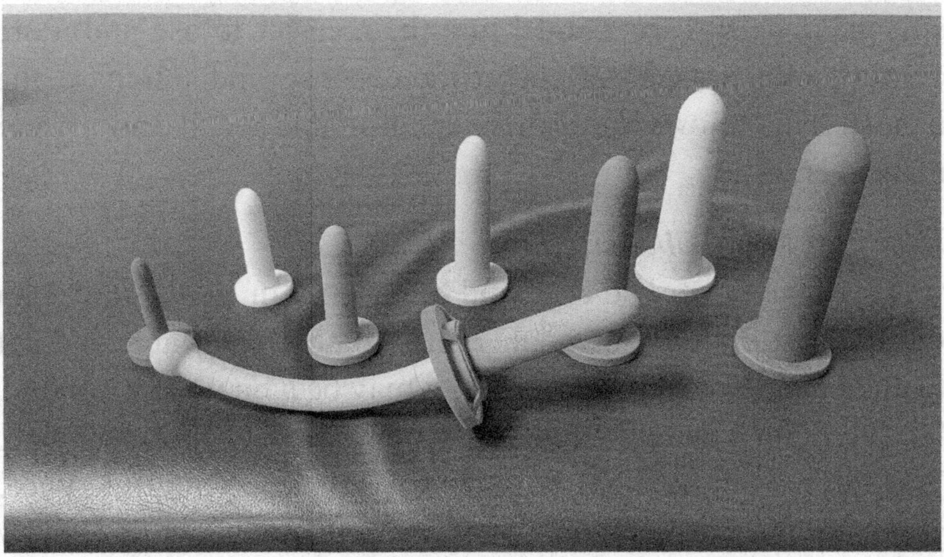

What is the goal of using a vaginal trainer?

The goal of a vaginal trainer is simple:

- Increase relaxation response of the pelvic floor muscles.
- Decrease muscular tension.
- Stretch the vagina and surrounding muscles in length and width.
- Aid in desensitizing the nervous system response by putting you in control of the speed and depth of penetration.
- Increase elasticity and capacity of the vagina.

What choices do I have?

There are actually quite a few choices, but the bottom line is to consider what they're made of. Typically, you'll find them in hard plastic or a softer medical-grade silicone options. Personally, I prefer the Intimate Rose brand and almost exclusively recommend their products. They're made of softer silicone and BPA free, and I find them easier to use and more comfortable. Spring for the extra expense and purchase the handle. This allows for a more comfortable reach and greater maneuverability.

How do I know what size to use?

If you've never had any kind of penetration at all, start with the smallest option. The goal is for it to be comfortable and not to elicit a pain response. Initially, it may be a bit uncomfortable, but anything beyond the thought of "annoying" is too much. We don't want to treat pain with pain. For your reference, you can look at the provider's website, but size one is usually comparable to a pencil. Size two is around the size of a woman's index finger. If you're already able to comfortably use regular or large tampons, start with size three. If you're already sexually active and just unable to accommodate your partner's size, you can bypass the smaller sizes. I suggest measuring your partner at full arousal and comparing that to the choices available. Start with a size or two below your goal and progress to the size of your partner if this is your goal. If you have not experienced any penetration, you will most likely want to purchase the smaller set (1–4) and as time progresses, purchase the next set (5–8). Of course, they can be purchased individually if the cost is prohibitive.

How long do I dilate and how often?

Duration: Studies indicate that 6–10 min is all you need. Other references out there may recommend longer but this is not necessary.

Frequency: Ideally use dilators three to four days per week. It is very important that you use a frequency that is within your comfort zone. The key to this and any self-care is consistency.

When to progress: Move to the next size when your trainer size is completely pain-free. Start with the previous size to warm up the tissue for a few minutes and then attempt to use the next size up.

What is the best position for using a vaginal trainer?

The position used previously for the wand is ideal. Be generous with the use of pillows for support. Don't forget you want your abdominal muscles and inner thigh muscles to be as relaxed as possible. Take time to relax and be comfortable.

How do I use a vaginal trainer?

As with the wand, wash with soap and warm water and dry to ensure a fresh start. Consider starting with a few minutes of hip stretches and some mindful breathing. Maybe even a nice little belly rub. Beginning with the wand is the perfect way to warm up the tissue, making it more receptive and relaxed. Three to five minutes should be plenty. If you do some preliminary warm-up activities, it should allow for ease of entry. Of course, you want to be free from distraction and not in a hurry.

- Set the stage in whatever fashion meets your needs. Apply a generous portion of water-based lubricant to the vaginal trainer and around the vaginal opening.
- Start with gentle pressure and slowly introduce the tip of the trainer to the vaginal opening. You may want to do some gentle reverse Kegels for an easier start. Some users find it helpful to do a few Kegels by using the contract/relax concept. Squeeze the pelvic floor muscles. Then, relax the muscles. Reattempt insertion to test for improvement.
- Ease your way into the vaginal canal. The larger flat end of the trainer remains outside the opening. Don't push forcefully or too quickly. The goal is to allow your body to accept the insertion without a tightening up of the pelvic floor muscles. Changing the pain-penetration pathway to the brain is the key to success.
- Insert the trainer straight in toward the spine or slightly downward. If you feel like you're hitting a wall, consider changing the angle. Everyone's canal has a slightly different angle, and just moving it a bit north or south can make a huge difference. Experiment with

different positions. Don't push straight up toward the belly button, as the urethra is located there and sensitive to pressure. Keep the trainer in place for six to ten minutes (even five can be beneficial if you're dealing with a time crunch). As you become more comfortable, introduce some movement—in and out, using various speeds as your comfort level allows. Getting used to the movement of the dilators in and out does, in the long run, make intercourse more comfortable. Feel free to try other positions that you might encounter during intimacy. Feel free as well to get your partner involved in any or all of these activities. It is helpful to open up the lines of communication and demonstrate what you are doing to address this. Get them to play along. I've found that many women experience pain when retracting the trainer for removal, so prepare yourself for this sensation. Use those reverse Kegels to release tension upon removal.

- Recent studies have indicated that practicing mindfulness techniques can be quite helpful while using vaginal trainers. Refer back to chapter 5 for some suggestions on calming the mind. Being distracted by watching TV or scrolling your phone is not suggested, as it takes you out of the present moment. Use positive affirmations that reaffirm the fact that you are doing something positive to improve your condition. Statements like: I am relaxed and at ease: I feel my body is comfortable and accepting this process: I am improving with each session: my vagina is open and receptive ... and, as always, remember to breathe!

Additional Options

VuVatech, in business since 2014, offers a viable alternative to the softer silicone option. They are the only patented vaginal trainers available with Neodymium magnets. Tara Langdale-Schmidt is the inventor, having suffered from pelvic pain herself. She combined her knowledge of the use of dilators with the science behind the use of magnets. Magnetic therapy has been around for years and is based on the premise that all living organisms exist in a magnetic field. And of course, the human body generates its own magnetic field. VuVa dilators contain over sixty strategically positioned core-based magnets that allow soothing energy to flow into the body, bringing fresh oxygenated blood to the surrounding nerves and muscles. For a list of studies regarding magnet therapy and results from clinical trials by Chief Investigator Dr. Michael Swor, see www.vuvatech.com.

In one study of eighteen women, the conclusions were such: "The VuVa magnetic dilator device is a safe and effective treatment of vulvovaginal pain. It performed significantly better than traditional vaginal dilators on standard pain tests."

Keep in mind that these are not to be used if you have a pacemaker, defibrillator, or any electrical device, or are pregnant or trying to become pregnant.

A Single Discrete Trainer

Milli, designed in conjunction with Stanford Biodesign engineers, top OB/GYNs, and pelvic physical therapist is the first product released by Materna Medical. This revolutionary technology was designed as an alternative to the static trainers, requiring up to eight different sizes. Designed of soft silicone and BPA free, including a vibrational option, this product adjusts incrementally (1 millimeter at a time from 15mm to 40mm) by touching a + or – button. This allows for expansion without the need to insert, remove, and reinsert various sizes. It was introduced to the market in 2017 and is getting favorable reviews. They received the Fast Company's "World-Changing Ideas" 2021 award for healthcare innovations. Take a look at www.milliforher.com to further explore this exciting option.

An Antimicrobial Option

BioMoi is in partnership with BioCote, a market leader in antimicrobial solutions. They have deliberately specified dilators made of U.S. Platinum Silicone, not plastic. This technology reduces microbes, such as bacteria, fungi, or viruses (preventing the growth of microorganisms), and minimizes product degradation. They are free of BPA, latex, and Phthalate. They're available in six sizes and are used in the same fashion as described above.

Lidocaine/Numbing Cream

This is a hot topic of debate among pelvic physical therapists. Some are in favor, and others are adamantly opposed. I've recommended it a handful of times. If you're finding it almost impossible or unbearable to use the wand or dilators, I do suggest that you give it a try. It isn't going to completely deaden the area, but it can take the edge off to allow for a little progress to be made. Sometimes, this is all it takes to get the ball rolling and have a win with the use of these tools. Obviously, the goal is to wean off the use of this cream but to get started, I personally don't see a problem with it. The maximum strength over the counter is 5 percent, and it can be purchased at any drug store. It's estimated that it takes approximately thirty minutes to become effective, and it lasts between thirty minutes and three hours.

I don't recommend the use of such creams for the purpose of intercourse. If you need this for penetrative intercourse, you're not ready to progress yet. Be patient and consistent with the tools described above, and the time will come. The key is consistency and commitment to the process. Stay positive and know that it will all be worth it in the end.

Looking for a plant-based option?

You may want to consider CBD vaginal suppositories. These are cannabis and hemp-based products. They are designed to enhance arousal and sexual intimacy. They ease discomfort for penetration and can be used in combination with vaginal trainers or prior to intercourse. Check out www.foriawellness.com, since 2014. They not only offer suppositories but an array of other products designed to enhance your satisfaction, comfort, and pleasure.

A Few Suggestions

- Keep in mind that depth isn't everything. Don't be concerned if you can't fully insert the trainer into the vaginal canal. Even partial insertion can be beneficial in stretching the more superficial pelvic floor tissue and in reframing the message to the brain about penetration.

- Feel free, as you get more comfortable, with the whole process to introduce movement inward and outward, mimicking intercourse. You can even practice doing a few Kegels with the dilator inserted if this is comfortable for you.
- Consider pulling the dilator partially out and stretching the tissue from 3:00 to 9:00, holding for 60–90 seconds in each position.
- Once you can actively insert and remove with no discomfort, it's time to move up to the next size.
- More lube is generally better. When you're ready to go up to the next size, it's recommended to start with the previous size to warm up the tissue prior to introducing the new size.
- Make sure you wash with soap and water and dry after each session and always keep clean and dry. If you're prone to urinary tract infections, urinate after each session.
- You may use a trainer when you're on your menstrual cycle. Just make sure that you clean thoroughly after each use.
- It's possible there could be some light vaginal bleeding when you first begin using dilators. If this persists, however, see your medical provider, as this isn't normal.
- Be patient with yourself. Don't get discouraged. Consistency is the key.
- If you feel like you need a break, you do! Listen to your body, and be your own best friend.

- Once you're able to be intimate with your partner with comfort, being together becomes your therapy. The body adapts to the demands. However, if there is a period of time that you are not being sexually active you may need to revisit using the trainers. Don't be disappointed. It's like taking a break from an exercise program.

The body is never the same from day to day. What worked yesterday may not work today. Just go with the flow, and as always ... remember to be kind to yourself. Exercise self-compassion with this and everything in life.

Real Stories from Real Patients: SM

Would you like to tell the readers a little about yourself?

I have always been incredibly active from sports to being outdoors. Living with vaginismus hindered my ability to do those things freely. I always suffered in silence and lived in shame dealing with this condition. I felt I couldn't talk to anybody about what was going on in fear of judgment and ridicule. How could something that is so natural like using a tampon or having sex hurt so much? I had so many failed relationships over the years and had never had a serious boyfriend as I feel like I always had a wall up with whoever I was dating. This condition was always in the back of my mind every day for as long as I can remember.

How long have you been dealing with this condition and what other treatments have you tried?

I have been dealing with this condition since I was around 16–17 when I discovered I could not tolerate the use of tampons due to extreme pain. I sought out help from my gynecologist at age 19 who asked if I had been sexually abused when I was a child as he believed that was the reason I was having pain. I told him no and asked him about a hymenectomy procedure and its benefits. I had a soccer teammate who told me she had the procedure done in high school as she was having pain with sex and tampon use. She told me after the procedure she was able to do those things pain-free. The result of the procedure ended up not working and the only information I had was that "anatomically I was fine." I continued to suffer in silence with this condition with failed relationship after failed relationship as I always felt I could not open up to the guy I was dating because this condition was always in the back of my mind. I was always missing out on beach trips with friends because I never knew if I would be on my period and had continued discomfort from pad use when playing soccer or working out. In the summer of 2020, I finally went back to the gynecologist but only because I was 26 and I had never had a successful pap smear and wanted to get screened for cervical cancer. Sure enough, I was unsuccessful once more however this time my physician had mentioned pelvic floor therapy. Long story short, I did not follow up with the therapist and I continued to suffer in silence until I had another failed relationship a year later in May of 2021. That's when I sought out help from my gynecologist and finally reached out to the pelvic floor therapist. I started my journey for pelvic floor therapy in July of 2021. During my first session, I could barely tolerate a manual exam by my therapist. My therapist had mentioned and ensure me that this is all done within my comfort zone and I was in control of the situation. It was uncomfortable to say the least, but it helped me have a better understanding of why I have this issue and ultimately how it can change.

Did you find the material/assignments easy to understand?

Yes, the assignments were easy to understand. My therapist really took the time to educate me on the various stretches and would show me the anatomy to help me get a better understanding. Every week she would add additional stretches and recommend different resources to read up on or purchase.

Did you find the assignments easy to implement? Why or why not? What were your biggest challenges and why?

My biggest challenge was the psychological component. Because I had such an intense pain in my pelvic region with any form of penetration, I never had the mind-body connection with my pelvic floor. This became such an issue and a hindrance in my progress that I was unable to use dilators as I had no familiarity with my own anatomy. It took me over 5 months of therapy before I was successful with my first dilator because I could not even look at my pelvic floor in a mirror! The anxiety I felt was so overpowering. My therapist continued to encourage me to begin the process of becoming familiar with my body before I tried the dilator again. That took the longest time for me and I did not think I would be able to get past the anxiety. Until I was finally successful with the first size dilator!

My second biggest challenge was not being able to lift weights, run, and do all my active things I had been so used to doing my whole life. I was incredibly active before starting therapy from lifting to playing soccer or frisbee to hiking. My therapist said on day 1 that if I want to be successful with this program I would have to put those things on pause. She did allow soccer once a week even though we had to compromise. But giving up those parts of my life was incredibly challenging, however, she told me that it is all temporary until I have completed my program and started seeing results.

What did you find was the easiest thing to do and why?

The easiest thing for me to do was the pelvic floor stretches. I am not a flexible person to begin with and doing those stretches every day helped me within my everyday life.

Would you recommend this treatment plan to others?

Yes, yes, yes. This treatment plan changed my life. I can only hope others out there have access to a therapist like I did because I do believe that is the key to why I was so successful.

How long did it take to start seeing results?

The results were slow but they happened at different stages. I noticed myself being able to relax my pelvic floor actively within the first couple of months. I began to see more results when my therapist implemented dry needling and felt more relaxation within my pelvic floor. But because I was not doing the dilators at home I feel as if my progress was hindered as I stated earlier. Once I got beyond the psych component and was able to use the dilators, my progress happened more quickly and I was able to progress from size 1 to size 3 and 4 within the first 2–3 months. I was successful with my first tampon in May of 2022. In June I was successful with my first pain-free pap smear. I feel as if I need to mention at this time I had been dating a guy for 5 months now. This was also a reason why I was motivated to use the dilators as this was one of the first guys I had told about my condition who did not run the other way. I also kind of liked this guy too! Fast forward to September of 2022, I was able to have pain-free sex for the first time in my life. The whole process took a little over a year. I also have been back to the gym and have transitioned back into my active lifestyle.

Would you like to add anything to help the readers better understand the process and what it takes to be successful?

This program works. Pelvic floor therapy works. I do believe I was so successful because I had such an amazing therapist who believed in me, was so knowledgeable as well as kind, and gave me tough love when I needed it. The first manual assessment she gave, I could barely tolerate. It brought me to tears for a number of reasons; physically, emotionally, and psychologically. A year later I can use tampons, have gynecology exams, and continue to have pain-free sex. I use the dilators as needed to supplement my active lifestyle. The only thing I regret was not starting this program sooner and not using the dilators sooner. Yes, you can just buy dilators but I do not believe you will be as successful. You have to have someone there to cheer you on, educate you, and perform the manual therapy needed to start the process.

7

The Mind-Body Connection

What happens when your body says yes but your mind says, whatever? I've always said, whatever is going on "up there" is going on "down there." We certainly cannot separate our mind from our body when it comes to our sexuality. In sex educator and author Dr. Emily Nagoski's book, Come As You Are: The Surprising New Science That Will Transform Your Sex Life, she speaks about arousal non-concordance. Simply put, this occurs when the brain and body are out of sync. This is more common than you can imagine and affects both men and women. It's also a completely natural part of our human sexuality. The sexual nature of our culture tells us that we should have this innate drive for sex and have it often. It tells us that as soon as we get aroused, our bodies should just stand up and take notice, and jump on board for the ride. The reality is that it's just not that simple. Sometimes, our body lags behind or may not get the clues at all. Or our brain is just not ready to let down the guard and take the next step. Rather than thinking there is something wrong with us, take some time and explore the information in Emily's book and listen to her Ted Talk. She gave a Ted Talk at TED2018 that covers this topic well. It's a master class in the science of sex that is appropriate for men and women. Her book is insightful, educational, and full of new research and theories that will open your mind to a new way of thinking about sexuality. She explains female sexuality in a way that is easily understood and thought-provoking. Her concept of introducing a sexual response that is driven by the gas and brake pedals is brilliant! No one teaches us this stuff! It's easy to see that we don't know what we don't know. She helps you understand your sexual temperament and the importance of context. This information is empowering and can open the door to a new sense of self and self-discovery. This book is highly praised. It's definitely on my recommended reading list.

Another outstanding author and veteran sex therapist, Dr. Bat Sheva Marcus, provides excellent resources in her book, Sex Points, Reclaim Your Sex Life with the Revolutionary Multi-Points System. It's a points-based system that empowers you to reach a richer understanding of your sexuality. She takes a look at 4 quadrants: Desire, Pain, Arousal, and Orgasm. Understanding her point system can bring things into a much clearer perspective and give you a better understanding of how these factors are all connected, ultimately affecting your experience of sexuality. When you purchase her book you also get free copies of The Pleasure Guide to Vibrators, The Pleasure Guide to Lubricants, and The Pleasure Guide to Bringing Sex Home Tonight. She provides a safe space to explore practical reasons that may be contributing to your disconnect and lack of satisfaction. If you go to her website, www.drbatsheva.com, you can sign up for her Newsletter and blog and take, free of charge, the Satisfaction Guaranteed Quiz. There's also information if you want to work with her directly including a free 10 min exploration session.

A July 14, 2022 article published by Oh-Nut, by writer and editor, Emma McGowan, a senior writer for an online privacy and security company, Avast, and former sex/relationship/dating writer at Bustle, presented information from a 2015 study out of the University of British Columbia. This study looked at, if teaching mindfulness practices would decrease sexual arousal non-concordance. This is a condensed version of the article.

Six Tips for More Mindful Sex

1. Focus on the process, not the outcome: Focusing on the outcome (a.k.a., the orgasm) can take you out of the present moment and disconnect the brain from the body. Instead, focus on what's happening to and in your body right NOW.
2. Practice in non-sexual settings: The therapist in the study had women practice mindfulness in areas that had nothing to do with sex for an entire month. They wanted them to really focus on being present in their bodies and in their lives in every aspect, from eating to driving...
3. Masturbate mindfully: This was the second piece of homework the sex therapist gave the participants. So many of us tune out from sex not only because we're distracted but because we were taught that sex is "dirty" or "bad." Our puritanical culture drills that message into us from a young age, and it can be really, really hard to move past it. Integrating mindfulness into masturbation can help push past that social conditioning.

4. Practice with a partner: The final piece of homework was to bring your mindfulness practice routine to the bed, car, couch, or shower with another person.
5. Breathe: This is Mindfulness 101 practice. It not only relaxes your body but brings your mind back to the present moment when it starts to drift. This might also give you clues about how aroused your body is at any given time.
6. Tune into other senses: Focus on touch, smell, sight, or taste. You might be surprised by how arousal shows up.

The Power of Thoughts

These conditions of vaginismus or arousal non-concordance can weight heavily on your mind. It can consume you—but only if you let it. In any case, though, thoughts are very powerful. They can lead you down the path of sadness and depression ... or that of hope and healing. First of all, I want you to let go of the idea that this will never get better—that you will always have this condition. Holding on to this mentality will only serve to keep you from moving forward in a positive direction.

As mentioned previously, most often once identified, understood, and treated, this condition generally improves. It's actually one of the easiest conditions to treat as a pelvic floor therapist. In fact, the success rate is huge! Hold on to this and believe it will improve. And if you need a little help in this department, consider cognitive behavior therapy (CBT) by finding a trusted professional in your area. Or seek a sex therapist that specializes in intimacy counseling.

Sometimes, we all need a little help. It's okay to admit that you can't walk this road alone. These professionals are there to guide you to a better way of thinking and provide tools that can be very helpful in overcoming your greatest fears and anxieties. And these days, it's easier than ever to find virtual options where you don't even have to leave the privacy of your home. One of my favorites in this area is Odela Health. Check out www.odelahealth.com for affordable sex coaching right in the privacy of your own home.

There's also another valuable resource available: namely, the Sounds True Foundation (www.soundstruefoundation.org). This organization is a 501(c)(3) creating equitable access to wisdom-based tools and practices. The foundation's creator, Tami Simon, has found a brilliant way of giving back. Her vision began in 1985 at the young age of twenty-two, and she has stayed true to "disseminating spiritual wisdom" over the years. The central focus is the practice of mindfulness and self-compassion. This is a lifeline she offers to others—one that's full of heart and hope. Her company, Sounds True Publishing, has released more than three thousand titles dedicated to spiritual wisdom. You can also access her information on her podcast, Sounds True: Insights at the Edge, where she interviews teachers and visionary writers.

Another priceless resource is the Mind Love Podcast. Host, Melissa Monte is one of today's most influential and thought-provoking explorers of the mindset and positive energy. She's a certified yoga instructor and Reiki healer. Her tagline is "Give your mind a little love today."

She always adds an element of humor and her own anecdotes, which often prove the most inspiring of all. She helps provide a mindset to help overcome some of life's biggest (and smallest) challenges. With two million downloads and counting, it's clear that she's on to something. So, don't miss out!

Real Stories from Real Patients: SR

Would you like to tell the readers a little about yourself?

I am 66 yrs old and have been looking for help for 30 yrs for chronic UTIs (always related to Intercourse) and painful intercourse. I went to several different gynecologists over the years and they would give me antibiotics. It was sad when you search on the computer and look for providers that are supposed to know this kind of thing but they just did not seem to have the answers. They just kept giving me antibiotics. Some even said, "You just have to suffer through this."

Can you imagine? I was shocked that treatment like this even existed and would love to have found this much earlier. It was amazing for me.

How long have you been dealing with this condition and what other treatments have you tried?

Literally for 30 years and the only option was medication and lubricant.

Did you have a positive outcome/were you pleased with the results and why?

Oh yes, I definitely had a positive outcome because it was like I was a real person again. It was great to have intimacy that I was no longer experiencing with my spouse. And of course, this made him happy as well.

Did you find the material/assignments easy to understand?

Yes. Even with the responsibility of traveling weekly to Gainsville to help care for my grandson, I was able to apply the principles and see the results I had hoped for.

Did you find the assignments easy to implement? Why or why not?

Very easy once I was shown the proper way to do them and given handouts. I learned never to cross my legs or do Kegels again. I had been doing Kegels since my first child was born decades ago, as every time I went to the doctor, they told me to do them. Little did I know that they were partially the cause of my problem.

What were your biggest challenges and why?

I had doubt that this would really work and was quite skeptical at first.

What did you find was the easiest thing to do and why?

Following up with the assignments at home.

Would you recommend this treatment plan to others?

100%.

How long did it take to start seeing results?

I saw results after 6 weeks and I only did my home program 2–3x a week but it worked.

Would you like to add anything to help the readers better understand the process and what it takes to be successful?

Come with an open mind and really dedicate yourself to following through on the assignments. It's worth the time and the effort.

8

You Got This!

Tenet 4: Fulfillment and Enjoyment

It's finally time to test the water and take the proverbial plunge! By this point, you've learned a lot about your body, the role that your central nervous system and mindset plays, and the tools out there to help you along your way. Hopefully, you feel empowered. If you've done the work and been dedicated to the process, then the rest should take care of itself. However, let's not ignore those last few pieces of the pelvic puzzle that will further serve to enhance your confidence. Let's inhale confidence and exhale doubt.

Four Phases of Sexual Arousal

According to Master and Johnson, the Sexual Response Cycle[6] is a model that categorizes sexual response into four phases and is the same for all genders.

[6]Masters WH and Johnson VE, (1966) Human Sexual Response, Boston MA: Little, Brown and Company

Phase 1: Excitement

This phase occurs in response to thoughts, sensations, or events that make someone feel aroused. This can be followed by an increase in heart rate, breathing, and blood pressure. There is typically increased muscle tension, blood flow to the genitals, erection for those who have a penis, and a start of lubrication for those who have a vagina.

Phase 2: Plateau

If sexual stimulation continues beyond the excitement phase, the second phase, a plateau is reached whereby the response that occurred during the first phase is further heightened. The vagina becomes more engorged with oxygen-rich blood, making it more receptive, expanding the walls, and elevating the uterus. This sounds like a good idea for anyone experiencing painful penetration—wouldn't you agree?

Phase 3: Orgasm

This occurs if the sexual stimulation continues beyond the plateau phase and leads to the peak of sexual excitement (i.e., "climax"). The pelvic floor muscles contract, creating a feeling of euphoria and a release of tension. The brain also releases a chemical called oxytocin (also known as the love hormone) and dopamine, which results in relaxation.

Phase 4: Resolution

In this phase, the body returns to the pre-aroused state. The heart rate, breathing, and blood pressure return to their normal levels. Typically, a person feels relaxed.

The Importance of Foreplay

It's no secret that men and women are wired differently on all levels, and sexual arousal is no exception. Men are genetically wired toward penetration. This is natural, as spreading their seed propagates the species. Women, on the other hand, typically view sex as more about intimacy, trust, and connection. As you can see in the phases described above, our body goes through a variety of changes from excitement to resolution. The importance of foreplay cannot be overlooked when dealing with vaginismus. It's often the key to unlocking the door to a happy and fulfilling sexual experience. Generally speaking, it does take a woman longer than a man to get aroused. It's safe to say, that most men are ready for penetration whenever they're at full erection. A woman's body doesn't respond that quickly. We're beautifully complex and have to respect this aspect of ourselves.

Foreplay helps us get in the mood mentally and moves us along the path of excitement physically. Once we're on that path mentally and emotionally, our body can follow. There are no rules here on how long or what type of foreplay is best. Everyone responds differently and likes different things. What's important is that you DO TAKE THE TIME FOR FOREPLAY!

Explore independently to see what you like and don't. The reality is that foreplay really begins with you. I often suggest that a woman take time, prior to being with her partner or spouse. Get in the right head space. Put on your favorite music, and light a candle. Do some juicy hip stretches and deep breathing. Even using the pelvic wand or vaginal trainer can be helpful to prestretch the superficial pelvic floor muscles. When it comes time to be together, get comfortable in communicating what feels good and, by all means, what doesn't. Let's take the mystique out of it and re-frame this. Think of it as "for play." It's about having a little fun together. Bring in some laughter and be lighthearted in the bedroom. Let your guard down and play together.

I think it's safe to say that we've all heard the term premature ejaculation, but while doing the research for this book, I came across the phrase "premature penetration." This was credited to a sex educator, Sheri Winston.[7] I think this is brilliant and deserves some thoughtful consideration. If the vagina is penetrated too quickly, without the proper time needed to promote expansion/lubrication and allow the uterus to rise, the end result will most likely be pain or at least the absence of pleasure.

Think about it another way: In the book, *The Pleasure Prescription*, A Surprising Approach to Healing Sexual Pain, one of the authors, Dee Hartmenn, PT, DTP, IF introduces the concept of 24/7 foreplay. Foreplay is the way you treat your partner on a daily basis. It's the tone of your voice, the little things you do for each other without expecting anything in return. It's going out of your way to promote the happiness and well-being of the person you cherish most. It's a mindfulness tactic in treating your partner with kindness, respect, and love on a daily basis and the payoff is enormous. Your relationship will be stronger, more fulfilling, and more joyful than ever before.

So don't ever let anyone tell you that foreplay is a waste of time or unnecessary. In fact, it's quite the opposite. Foreplay is

---

[7]Sheri Winston, Woman's Anatomy of Arousal: Secret Maps to Buried Pleasure Kingston NY Margo Garden Press 2010

of paramount importance, and by practicing a mindful approach to foreplay you are creating a foundation of love and respect that will last a lifetime that goes far beyond the bedroom.

Looking For a Great Place to Start?

Consider something called, Sensate focused touch. It was developed by Dr. William Masters and Dr. Virginia Johnson in the 1960s. The goal is to open lines of communication to create intimacy and take the focus away from the performance anxiety. It's more about the connection, not the orgasm. It is described as mindful touch or non-orgasmic touch. The original techniques can be summarized in a five-step process:

Step 1—Non-genital touching: This focuses more on the soft, sensual nature of touch, not the sexual nature. It's about touching and being touched. It's designed to reduce sexual anxiety and provide opportunities to just explore each other's bodies. Start out when you are both in a restful, relaxed state. Take time to prepare a conducive space. Get comfortable and spend 10–15 min exploring each other's bodies taking turns. Do not focus on touching the genital area. This is to be done as an experience that promotes the pure sensory level of touch, without any expectation of an outcome. Take time to get to know each other's bodies.

Step 2—Genital/breast touching: This is similar to Step One but there are no off-limits areas this time. But again, the experience should focus on exploration, not necessarily sexual stimulation. It is encouraged to guide the partner doing the touching to direct them to the right spots and increasing or decreasing the pressure that is being applied.

Step 3—Adding lotion or massage oil: Similar to step 2 but add the medium to facilitate a gliding/sliding on the tissue to enhance the experience.

Step 4—Mutual touching: Here both partners are in unison to touch one another at the same time. As with the other steps, it is suggested not to use this with the intention of sexual arousal but to further enhance the experience of exploration. Use of the tongue is permitted but kissing or oral sex is not encouraged.

Step 5—Sensual Intercourse: Masters and Johnson were very intentional in naming this last step.

The goal is to enrich the experience of touch, by increasing the level of awareness. It's important to use all the senses of sight, smell, sound, and touch. It's all meant to open up the lines of communication and ultimately feel a deeper sense of connection.

Depending on where you are in your intimacy journey or experience, these exercises can be done over the course of weeks or months in getting to know each other. Or they can be done sequentially leading you both down the path of arousal, fulfillment, and connection.

Want to Find Out Your Bedroom Personality?

If you're a NETFLIX fan, you may have seen or heard about Gwyneth Paltrow's Sex, Love, and Goop, which references the Erotic Blueprint Types by somatic sexologist, author, and public speaker, Miss Jaiya. You can take the Erotic Blueprint Quiz to see what your bedroom personality is or dive deeper and take her Erotic Blueprint Breakthrough Course. These tools are another means to enhance your understanding of what you like and don't. They can further advance your confidence to have the best sex of your life and look forward to intimacy, rather than considering it just another obligation, or another thing on your "to-do" list. In Jaiya's own words: "I believe that sex isn't something we do. Sex is essential to our health, our vitality, and vibrant aliveness." She and her partner, Ian, have created quite a buzz in the world of sexuality. Check out these valuable resources at www.missjaiya.com.

Lotions, potions, and devices, oh my!

Lube Is a Girl's Best Friend! (Seriously!)

We naturally produce lubrication from our Bartholin glands and the cervix during sexual arousal. This reduces friction during penetration and can be a key factor in addressing pain. It also reduces the chances of vaginal tears, which can lead to more serious issues like infections and a higher risk of sexually transmitted diseases. What you may not know is that it's common, even among healthy individuals, for this lubricant to be insufficient. The use of lubricant doesn't in any way indicate that you're not interested in your partner. Low production of lubrication can occur due to certain medications, hormonal changes during pregnancy, after childbirth, while nursing, or during menopause. "A 2009 study from Indiana University of 2453 women reported in 70% of events, women indicated that using lubricant made sex feel very pleasurable and more comfortable (65.5%)."[8]

---

[8]Studies about "Why Men and Women Use Lubricants During Sex" Nov 9, 2009, Indiana University Science Daily

If you take a trip down any drugstore aisle or look on the Internet, the choices can be confusing and a bit overwhelming. Before you buy, know to avoid lubricants that contain artificial flavors, colors, sugars, essential oils, additional additives, or glycerin. Avoid anything with a "warming sensation" as this can be more than you bargain for and downright unpleasant once applied. Look for things like parabens, sulfates, or propylene glycol. All of these should be avoided as well. Check the ingredients and look at reviews. Remember our vaginas have a natural bacterial flora and certain products may alter this balance or change the pH. If you're sensitive, I suggest a wrist test first. Here are some of your options:

Water-Based – These are the most natural-feeling lubes and may be the best initial choice if you're concerned about additives. Try to pick one with a pH of around 3.8 to 4.5 to reduce the risk of altering your balance. These products are safe to use with silicone sex toys, dilators, or wands. However, it does dry out quickly and often needs to be reapplied.

Silicone-Based – These lubricants are usually hypo-allergenic and often used by those with skin sensitivity or allergies. They usually last longer and can be used in water. Though they can be a bit sticky, their longer-lasting effects are often worth it. Not to be used with silicone sex toys, dilators, or wands, as they break down the materials.

Hybrid – These lubricants are a blend of oil and water—typically 90 percent water-based.

Oil-Based – These are the most commonly used lubricants and my personal favorite, as they're longer-lasting and natural (organic cold-pressed coconut oil, olive oil, etc.).

Very Important: Oil-based lubricants are not to be used with latex and some non-latex condoms or diaphragms. Some lubricants may affect sperm function, potentially decreasing the chances of pregnancy.

Companies to Consider

- www.ahyes.org – Certified organic products designed to be side-effect free, natural, and pH-matched to the vagina.
- www.goodcleanlove.com CEO, Wendy Strgar is an author, sex educator, and loveologist. She is a writer of an award-winning blog, Making Love Sustainable. She is also the author of two books: Sex That Works: An Intimate Guide to Awakening Your Erotic Life and Love that Works: A Guide to Enduring Intimacy. They even have a fertility-friendly option.
- Desert Harvest Aloe Glide 100% natural Aloe Vera based.

How to Apply and Insert

Have a hand towel or washcloth nearby to use for your hands after applying. Use the product generously on the penis, covering it from the base to the tip. Have fun with it and make it pleasurable for both of you. Put a little on the vaginal opening as well. Don't be shy! Reapply! This next point is of utmost importance, so take notice! I highly recommend that you take control of your partner's penis when it comes to insertion. If you take matters into your own hands (what a pun), it will give you a sense of control that is often needed in this situation. Go slow, take some nice long deep breaths, and do some reverse Kegels. Try different positions. There are some great suggestions in the Women's Health article by Nicole Blades, Aryelle Siclait, Sabrina Talbert and Marissa Gainsburg published October 24, 2022: Add These 49 Best Sex Positions To Your Bedroom Bucket List. By all means, communicate with your partner. Believe me, he wants to hear from you and how he can make this easier. And, speaking from personal experience I can tell you that often if you can get past the vaginal sphincter muscle, the bulbocavernosus which is often tight, as it should be naturally, you are home-free. The pain is usually very short-lived and the pleasure that follows is seconds away.

Fun in the Bedroom or Wherever!

Toys aren't just for kids anymore, and they definitely aren't just for single women. They can be a perfect addition to turn up the heat in any situation. Let go of the shame or embarrassment regarding the idea of using a toy. It's time to be open-minded and consider this all-important addition to your sexual experiences. Using a sex toy can improve intimacy and enhance your relationship. It opens the lines of communication up to talk about what feels good and brings pleasure. It's recommended to be used during foreplay and most importantly during penetration. Clitoral stimulation is key to sexual satisfaction and a toy is the perfect tool to get that all-important area of excitement that's just screaming for attention. Consider visiting a local sex shop. Make a date for it. These places are there to enhance your pleasure and enjoyment. They aren't sleazy or dirty. They're full of every kind of toy you can imagine (or can't imagine). The staff is usually very friendly and helpful. They've heard it all and certainly won't judge!

If that's not your cup of tea, though, go online and take a look at what's available. The options are many. All of these toys are scientifically designed to aid in your sexual experience. They're created for the human body and intended for pleasure. So whether you want an external vibrator or an internal vibrator, take a deep dive and see what you can find. It may surprise you! Three that are high on the radar and easy to incorporate into your time together: a cock ring, the rose toy, and a bullet vibrator. They are external. The cock ring is a handy little addition that provides pleasure for both parties, and there is no better way to stimulate the clitoris during penetration than the cock ring. I promise! Like the ring, the vibrating bullet is small and convenient to use for clitoral stimulation during penetration as well. Its small size can easily be manipulated to be used in multiple positions without interference. The rose toy has numerous options to explore as well. And if you are looking for a toy to stimulate the G-Spot, among others areas of interest, check out POCO by Soul Source. It's easily adjustable and can be bent into different shapes. Go ahead and take the plunge. You have very little to lose and a ton of fun to gain!

A San Francisco author and medical journalist that takes a look at this subject in Sizzling Sex for Life: How to Maximize Erotic Pleasure at Any Age (2021) is Michael Castleman, MA. He posted a blog in Psychology Today on March 16, 2009, with over 50 million views. "It's perfectly normal for women not to have an orgasm during intercourse. Most women need direct clitoral stimulation to experience orgasm. Intercourse simply doesn't provide enough direct clitoral stimulation to allow most women to become aroused enough to have orgasms." Michael answers questions about sex and sexuality for free on the site he hosts: www.greatsexguidance.com.

Lotions and Potions to Address Vaginal Dryness

Vaginal dryness can occur at any age due to the use of birth control pills, cancer treatment, post-surgery, menopause, breastfeeding, or postpartum effects. The loss of estrogen can play havoc on the vaginal wall and vulva. This occurs before, during, and after menopause. This is a time when the walls of the vagina become thinner and less elastic. This is the medical term for vaginal atrophy and is probably the number one reason for painful intercourse in women over forty.

Hormone-Free Options

There is a growing interest in a non-hormonal alternative to treating vaginal dryness/tissue health. Hyaluronic acid (HA), discovered in 1934, is a naturally occurring substance in our bodies that serves to conserve and protect water molecules in the skin cells. You may be familiar with this, as it's often found in anti-aging products for the face. Its purpose is to keep our tissues lubricated and moist. Its popularity is increasing in a multitude of products. One such product is used to treat vaginal dryness. HA has known properties to aid in addressing dryness and retaining moisture. This product is typically delivered in a cream form directly into the vaginal canal with a plastic applicator or via suppositories 2–3 times per week. A 2013 study compared HA with estrogen and found it to be as effective.[9]

---

[9]Is vaginal hyaluronic acid as effective as vaginal Estriol for vaginal dryness relief Retra State Arch Gynecol Obstet 2013, Dec 288 (6) 1199-201

Products to Consider

- BioNourish from Goodcleanlove
- Revaree from Bonafide
- Silk, Silver, or Gold by Neueve (you can take a quiz to see what's right for you)
- Hyalo Gyn
- RepaGyn
- Gynatrof

Or you can see your health care provider for a referral/RX to a compounding pharmacy.

Products for External Use

The external labia can get dry and the incidence of labia skin tears is not uncommon. Consider the following for external use:

- #1 on the list is Julva at drannacabeca.com. This product rejuvenates vaginal tissue, restores moisture, prevents bladder leaks, intensifies sensation, and improves skin elasticity.
- Vmagic vulva care and Intimate skin cream by Medicine Mama
- Ahyes VB
- JoyLux Revitalize HER
- Organic cold pressed Coconut oil

A Device Worthy of Recognition

There's a great little company out of Seattle Washington with a premium line of products made by women for women called JoyLux. The founder, Colette Courtion, and Dr. Sarah de la Torre, MD, DIPABLM have partnered together to provide cutting-edge science to address intimate wellness in a way no other company has. Their products are hormone free, clean, and pH-balanced. But their intimate wellness device, V-Fit Gold is epic!!! It uses LED (red and near-infrared), vibration, and heat to stimulate collagen and increase nitric oxide. This device is designed to be used at home, synced to an app on your phone, and provides ongoing support to vaginal tissue. They have been featured in/on Allure, Goop, NewBeauty, and Vogue. See www.joylux.com for their unique story and studies backed by science—definitely worth the investment and the time! Their mission is "to empower women to live confidently by improving all aspects of their intimate health." They have even gone a step beyond their original mission to bring a new product to the market just for new moms who have experienced a vaginal tear during delivery. In April 2023, Mommy Matters was created. Their newest product, NEO HEAT; Repair the Tear offers this innovative red and infrared LED light to give new mommies fast, effective relief. If you are suffering from a post-vaginal delivery tear, make sure to check out this valuable resource.

Other Medical Treatment Options

Any web search regarding pelvic floor dysfunction may lead you to information about the use of Botox injections, the O-Shot, or dry needling. Botox is commonly used at medical spas to address facial wrinkles and such, but they're also used in the treatment of vaginismus. This procedure is designed to decrease muscle tension and reduce excessive muscle activity. Typically administered by pain-management physicians, Botox is injected directly into the pelvic floor muscles. As of 2020, Botox isn't FDA-approved for pelvic floor dysfunction. However, data shows that its use in this area is promising.

The O-Shot, marketed as the orgasm shot, is a non-surgical procedure to increase sexual arousal and rejuvenate the vagina. Unlike Botox, the O-Shot uses PRP (plasma-rich protein) spun down from your own blood. It's injected directly into the clitoris and labia. Some women claim the treatment improves their orgasm experience but there is no rigorous scientific evidence that the O-Shot works as promised. This isn't meant to treat an overactive pelvic floor which is typically found in the condition of vaginismus.

Dry needling is delivered by a physical therapist trained in this technique. Some states allow physical therapists to use acupuncture needles for the delivery of treatment directly into the muscles. This can be a very effective addition to the other techniques that a pelvic floor therapist would typically use to treat an overactive pelvic floor. Believe it or not, the procedure, if delivered skillfully, isn't painful, but of course, every patient has their own sensitivities and thresholds.

Last but Not Least

This section isn't intended to be a substitute for professional medical advice, diagnoses, or treatment. This is for general information only, and as always, do your own research and speak with your medical provider.

When estrogen runs low, the effects can be many. Some of the most common are vulvar/vaginal atrophy, inflammation of the vagina (atrophic vaginitis), and inflammation of the urethra (atrophic urethritis). According to the National Women's Health Network, "as research stands, it appears that vaginal estrogen is a safe and effective treatment for vaginal discomfort due to menopause and has a much lower risk of the cancers and cardiovascular events typically associated with hormone therapy."

The Women's Health Initiative Observational Study showed that for "women with an intact uterus, who used vaginal estrogen, the risks of stroke, invasive breast cancer, colorectal cancer, endometrial cancer, pulmonary embolism/deep vein thrombosis were not significantly different between vaginal estrogen users and nonusers."[10] If you're considering this option, it's recommended that you speak to your healthcare provider, and if you experience vaginal bleeding once the process begins, see your doctor immediately, as this could be a sign of an overgrowth of the lining of the uterus (the endometrium).

Note: Bioidentical hormones such as Estradiol (E2) and Estoril (E3) are plant-based and have the same molecular structure as the hormones made by your body. Synthetic hormones such as Premarin and Vagifem don't, but your body converts them to usable forms. Regardless of which route you may be considering, both require a prescription from a physician and are not available over the counter. If you need to consult with an online provider, consider www.odelahealth.com—a digital health clinic that supports women throughout every chapter of their sexual journey from postpartum to menopause and beyond.

As you can see, there are numerous options to address concerns regarding vaginal dryness and atrophy. Take a

[10]The Journal of North American Menopause Society Jan 2018 Volume 25 Issue 1 p 11-20
Original article: Breast cancer, endometrial cancer, and cardiovascular events who used vaginal estrogen in the Women's Health Initiative Observational Study Crandall, Carolyn J, MD, MS, et al

little time and research these yourself and speak to your provider. As always, be patient and open to trying more than one option to find what works best for you and your body. Keeping a journal may be helpful—and remember to always follow the manufacturer's recommendations.

Real Stories from Real Patients: RH

How long have you been dealing with this condition and what other treatments have you tried?

I knew something wasn't quite right because I'd never been able to use tampons without pain. I didn't try to address the problem until I was engaged though. I was 25 and saw my GYN for a 1st pap smear, which was almost intolerable, but was told that was likely because I wasn't used to things happening down there and would adjust with time. Once I got married I realized it was a bigger problem than I thought. My husband and I are both missionaries. I was a virgin when we got married. I knew it was going to be rough, but was not prepared for the disappointment I was met with on our honeymoon. We tried a few exercises found in some popular Christian sex books (which did not at all discuss women's pain with sex beyond a mild discomfort the 1st time), such as slowly inserting fingers and stretching until you reach the size of a penis, to no avail. It was so incredibly painful and I was devastated. We found other ways of being intimate and my husband was so kind and understanding. About 8 months later (I waited that long because I was not convinced that anyone would be able to do anything to help me) I went back to the same GYN, who then diagnosed me with vaginismus and sent me to Sandi.

Did you have a positive outcome/were you pleased with the results and why?

Yes! I was very skeptical at the start of PT and pretty anxious as well. It's an extremely vulnerable position to be in, both physically & mentally. I remember a few times, in the beginning, leaving so discouraged and sore, thinking that there was no way this would ever get better. But after about 6 months, I graduated and am now able to use tampons and have penetrative sex with my husband, which was the goal of PT for me.

Did you find the material/assignments easy to understand?

Yes, I felt that things were well explained and helpful both in overcoming pain as well as growing in knowledge of my own anatomy.

Did you find the assignments easy to implement? Why or why not?

For the most part, yes. The difficulty was finding time to do them. It can feel like a lot to suddenly implement into your routine but it is definitely worth the time.

What were your biggest challenges and why?

I think my biggest challenges were mental. I was so discouraged and felt like such a failure after my honeymoon when we were not able to be intimate in the way I had imagined. I wanted to work toward getting better but was so discouraged and often doubted that anything was going to help. It was so helpful to have someone (Sandi) who was encouraging and rooting for me.

What did you find was the easiest thing to do and why?

Implementing the recommended stretches was definitely the easiest because that didn't directly involve the areas of my body where I was experiencing pain.

Would you recommend this treatment plan to others?

100% yes. Anyone experiencing any level of pain with penetration, whether from intercourse or tampon use, should pursue pelvic floor physical therapy.

How long did it take to start seeing results?

Maybe after about 10–12 visits. I think that was about the time that I was instructed to start using dilators and I remember being pretty scared of that but shocked at how easy it was. I think that was when I started to feel more encouraged and to believe that this really could work.

Would you like to add anything to help the readers better understand the process and what it takes to be successful?

The biggest thing for me was consistency, both in going to PT and in doing the recommended exercises. I didn't do this well and I imagine my process could have gone faster if I had.

9

The Clit Is It!

In case you wondering, the last chapter is about ONE thing and ONE thing only: the Clitoris! Yes, it has a chapter all its own—that's how essential it is. One relevant thing that you may not know is that it's estimated that only 25 percent of women are able to consistently reach orgasm during penetrative intercourse. Yes, I said 25 percent! Sounds shocking, right? This statistic comes from thirty-three studies over the past eighty years by Elisabeth A. Lloyd, an American philosopher of biology and professor, and can be further understood in her book The Case of the Female Orgasm (Harvard University Press). On the flip side of this coin, 96% of men reach orgasm with penetration. What's wrong with these statistics? Why have women not been educated about this information? Why don't we know this? I believe the answer lies in the power of the clitoris. It's time we stand up and take notice of this knowledge, embracing the power from within. It's time we start talking about this to one another and to our partners. It's time to start having this collective conversation.

Get Cliterate

It seems that pleasure and the clitoris are finally getting some much-deserved limelight. However, it was not until 1998 that an Australian urologist and professor, Dr. Helen O'Connell finally uncovered just how large the clitoris actually is. It makes you wonder what took so long In 2005, she shed some astounding light on this little gem, which isn't so little after all, in Anatomy of the Clitoris. She actually did some micro dissections on cadavers and looked at MRIs of real women. She compares the clitoris to an iceberg and discovered an entire clitoral complex. Internally, it's ten times larger and estimated to be at least the size of the average penis. It boasts 8000+ nerve endings and is the only known body part whose sole purpose is to give pleasure. Don't you think this insight in itself is enough reason to explore and befriend this part of your body? You can view Dr. Oconnel's TEDx Talks on Sept 15, 2020, Get Cliterate. There's also a fascinating YouTube video by Scientific America, It Took 2000 Years to Find the Clitoris. This 8-minute video, by Rachel E. Gross, an award-winning science journalist, covers the history of the anatomy and its more recent discoveries. Her book, Vagina Obscura, was released in 2022 and chosen as the New York Time Editor's Choice and The Best Science Book of 2022 by Smithsonian and Science News.

The glans clitoris is what most people refer to as the clit. This is a small nodule just beneath the clitoral hood, which is the apex where the labia minora meet.

Just beneath the glans is the corpora (body), which branches into two legs down toward the vaginal opening, known as the crura. These form a V from the urethra to the vaginal opening.

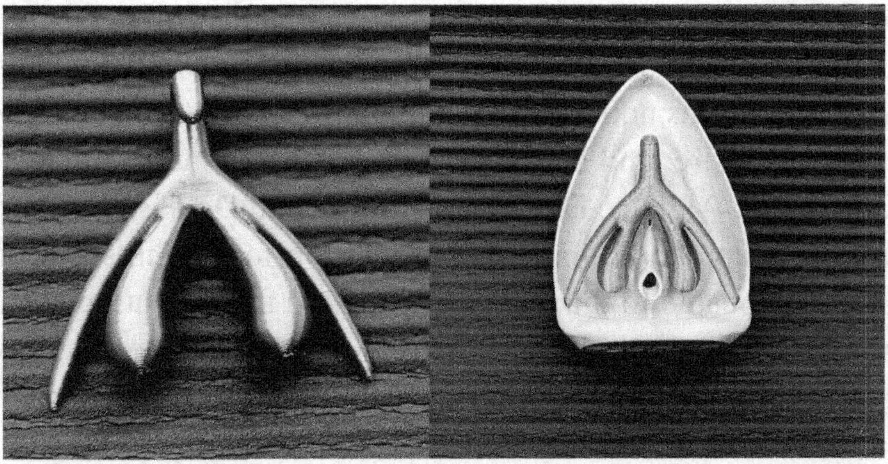

Between the vaginal wall and the crura are the vestibular bulbs, which engorge with blood during arousal. At the joining point of the crura is the root. Since the clitoris is protected by the labial lips and the hood, it's necessary to gently press the hood upward and part the lips to find the sensitive glans, which is the most important area for sexual pleasure. It's often referred to as the shape of an inverted flower. Learning how to find the clitoris and knowing how to stimulate it can make all the difference in the world in sexual intimacy or self-pleasure.

Anatomical Art

Interested in seeing an artist's rendition of the clitoris? Explore the work of Sophia Wallace, an American conceptual artist and photographer: 100 Natural Laws of Cliteracy. It's a text installation created in 2012, the first in an ongoing project. It "upholds that all bodies are entitled to pleasure, which is fundamental for full citizenship."

Her TEDxSalford talk is also enlightening: "A Case for Cliteracy." Visit her website to see her work, a link to her speeches, and the documentary released in 2020 called Dilemma of Desire. This movie explores the work of four women who are shattering myths and lies that women are being told about their sexuality, desire, and bodies. It's directed by Maria Finitzo and stars Sophia Wallace, Dr. Stacey Dutton, and Dr. Lisa Diamond. I certainly applaud Sophia on her passion for this mission. She is truly dedicated to this body of work and the education of men and women about this long-over-do lesson in female anatomy.

www.sophiawallace.art.com for this and more amazing (clitoral) content!

Know Thyself

If you haven't explored this very extraordinary, exquisite, and highly sensitive part of your body, it's never too late. Or did you explore this erogenous zone when you were a little girl, finding it quite delightful, but got the message that it was a forbidden pleasure? Perhaps it's time to reconnect with that little girl and find that delight again. So, take a deep breath and let go of the embarrassment or shame that hundreds of years of misleading societal messages have placed upon us. It's time to remove this heavy burden from our collective shoulders about these oppressive cultural messages. Allow yourself to explore this very special part of your body that is solely there for your pleasure. Exploring your own sensuality can open your senses to a whole new way of being. It's about giving yourself permission to feel good, and isn't it about time? Let's embrace this idea of cultivating sensuality within and FOR ourselves. Once we cultivate it, it can permeate into other aspects of our life making us feel more playful, happy, and fulfilled. This isn't just about sexuality, it's about being present in your body. It's about a deeper sense of embodiment, that transcends us to a deeper connection within. It's tuning into your sense of sight, sound, smell, taste, and touch. Sensuality is about getting in touch with your body and your own femininity. It really is a superpower that lies deep within each of us but we have to take the time to explore it. Finding the divine feminine within is like a hidden treasure, just waiting patiently to be found. It allows us to remember who we are. It can be a portal into a deeper sense of self. I have always loved the question, who are you becoming? It is a lifelong question that we must continue to ask ourselves. After all, the journey of self-discovery is ongoing and it has the power to unleash undiscovered gifts of creativity, build confidence, and foster intimacy with ourselves. This inner resource can have profound benefits that have been untapped, until now…

Start with some simple things that help you develop a deeper sense of self-confidence and exploration just for you. You deserve to tap into your inner resource and unleash the profound benefits that come with exploring your sensuality:

- Take a hot bath with all the bells and whistles (music, candles, essential oil, or bubbles)
- Get a massage or facial
- Buy yourself some new underwear, bra, or pajamas that make you feel good inside
- Buy a sexy new dress or those shoes you've had your eye on
- Get that great haircut you've always wanted to try
- Try a more daring shade of lipstick that you think looks so great on everyone

- Walk through the house naked
- Learn to belly dance or take salsa lessons
- Read a romance novel or some erotica
- Buy a piece of sculpture or a piece of art that reminds you of your sensual/feminine side
- Dance like no one is watching to your favorite music

If you need a little more prompting, check out, New York sex and relationship therapist, Dr. Megan Fleming and The Pleasure Challenge, a free nine-day program with exercises to keep pleasure at the top of your list, rather than the bottom. www.greatlifegreatsex.com.

For some in-depth reading to help you tap into the power within, check out a powerful essay by Audre Lorde; Uses of the Erotic: The Erotic as Power. She has left behind a powerful legacy of speeches and essays that has influenced feminist thinking for years.

When you are ready to do some more in-depth exploration, first of all, take the time to create a safe space to explore and see what feels good to you. This time of self-discovery is paramount in getting to know yourself. We have to stop turning away from the "YES" within ourselves. If you don't know what you like, how can you communicate this to another? Don't be shy. This really is the key to unlock your pleasure. Start with some lubricant to avoid friction. Start slow and soft with some gentle circular movements, tapping, or up-and-down massage. Use a mirror if you really want to see what you're doing. Try lightly pinching it or using a toy—even the spray from the shower head. Since we know that a large part of the clitoris extends into the vaginal canal, penetration may offer that added excitement you're looking for. Refer back to the section on toys and consider adding one to your discovery journey. They offer an element of stimulation that your own fingers don't have. The takeaway here is that you shouldn't underestimate the power of the clitoris. And yes, it can be said that you hold the key to pleasure and orgasm at the tip of your fingers.

The Ever-Illusive G-Spot (Named After Dr. Ernst Grafenberg)

We cannot have a conversation about female anatomy without a discussion regarding the almighty and somewhat illusive G-Spot. It's said to be found fully inside the vagina. This was introduced by Dr. Beverly Whipple, PhD, RN, FAAN-AASECT, a certified sex educator and researcher after she discovered the motion used to beacon someone to "come here" inside the vagina, produced a strong response in some women. This spot isn't as easy to discover at the clit. "In a 2017 study, researchers attempted to find this spot and actually came up empty-handed."[11] The recent theory states that it may actually be an area consisting of five zones that make up part of the clitoral network: the clitoral crura, the clitoral bulb, the Skene's gland (located on each side of the urethra), the urethra, and the front wall of the vagina. Some women claim that a G-spot orgasm is stronger than that of a clitoral orgasm, but there is little evidence to support this claim.

[11]The Journal of Sexual Medicine The "G-Spot" is Not a Structure Evident on Marcoscopic Anatomic Dissection of the Vaginal Wall; Nathan HoagMD, FRCSC Ja et R Keast PhD, Helen E O'Connell MD, MBBS, FRACS 2017. 10.071

Real Stories from Real Patients: SL

Would you like to tell the readers a little about yourself?

I'm a 30-year-old woman who was recently married. When my husband and I started to discuss getting pregnant, it surfaced a conversation about my body that I've been putting off for a while. As a teenager, I had a tailbone injury that never healed (I've been experiencing chronic pain for 15 years!), intercourse had pain in different areas and I wasn't sure what to do about it. My OBGYN recommended physical therapy that specialized with the pelvic floor—so I did!

How long have you been dealing with this condition and what other treatments have you tried?

Altogether, I've had pain for 15 years.

Did you have a positive outcome/were you pleased with the results and why?

Absolutely! The pain is no longer chronic and I now have the tools to continue to heal the different parts of my pelvic area.

Did you find the material/assignments easy to understand?

Definitely. The building blocks of the treatment were methodical, clear, and comprehensive. I learned that this therapy is physical work paired with emotional/mental parts.

Did you find the assignments easy to implement? Why or why not?

The stretches were easy to implement and super effective. The pelvic wand definitely had a learning curve, but Sandi and Danielle were great about teaching me how to effectively use it on my own during in-office sessions. They even gave me instructions for my husband to help out with at-home therapy.

What were your biggest challenges and why?

The challenge was the process itself. Dealing with pain that you've had for over a decade is difficult to push through. Physical therapy showed me that the pain I was experiencing was way deeper rooted in my body than I thought. The techniques that were needed were initially scary, but Sandi and Danielle were the most compassionate and made me feel comfortable the entire time.

What did you find was the easiest thing to do and why?

The stretches! Although some of them required some conditioning, they were not complicated and were a welcomed addition to my at-home routine.

Would you recommend this treatment plan to others?

HELL YES. I think especially people with uteruses need to experience this form of physical therapy. Society has dismissed our pain and conditioned us that it's okay not to know what's happening with this part of our bodies. The emotional and mental connections we have in this part of our bodies are incredible and developing that care and awareness for it is so so important. I know this deeply now. I love my pelvic floor and care for it now that I know how to. You will be amazed what you learn about yourself.

How long did it take to start seeing results?

Of the 5 months of therapy, I started seeing results within a month.

Would you like to add anything to help the readers better understand the process and what it takes to be successful?

As a woman with a uterus and a period, I genuinely thought the pain and mystery of my pelvic floor and all its connected parts were normal. Doctors dismissed my tailbone pain for 15 years. Pain with intercourse was something I "powered through." I honestly had no idea what was even possible with this kind of physical therapy and what techniques were even available. This part of my body is sensitive and requires the discussion of sensitive topics (intercourse, access through the rectal canal, etc) so even though the mechanics of this therapy was great, I don't think I would have gotten the results I did without the equally important compassion from Sandi and Danielle. They were equal parts encouraging me to push limits for progress and made sure that I was comfortable every step of the way. I literally tell all my friends about this process.

A Few Parting Thoughts

As I come to the end of this book, I reflect on the profound impact this journey has had on me as a woman, a therapist, and a seeker of the truth. It has been a personal pilgrimage that has led me to this moment, fueled by a deep desire to help women, just like you who suffer from this all-too-common condition. My hope is that this guidebook serves as a beacon of hope—a light that shines through the darkness. In it, I hope that you have found the answers to addressing the pain that has kept you in despair and stopped you from enjoying something as beautiful as your sexuality and sense of sensuality. I have spent countless hours researching and pondering—praying that this guidebook will provide a healing balm to a deep wound that affects so many. As you know all too well, this condition is often not discussed openly with others. It carries with it embarrassment, shame, and guilt. It's painful on so many levels, affecting the mind, the body, and the spirit.

Well, no more! May your mind be at ease knowing that you hold the key to happiness in the palm of your hand. May your body finally enjoy pleasure beyond your wildest imagination. And may your spirit soar with a new level of freedom and fulfillment when you claim victory! It has been an honor to guide you on this journey toward a brighter, more fulfilling future.

"I am not free while any woman is unfree, even when her shackles are very different from my own."—Audre Lorde

At a Glance

1. Don't be so hard on yourself.
2. When in doubt, Breathe.
3. Relax your belly and your jaw.
4. Trust the process. It works.
5. Stay calm under pressure. Remember, it's all a pressure system.
6. Speak your truth with love and compassion.
7. Explore and befriend your clitoris.
8. Use lube … generously.
9. Use toys and have some fun.
10. Smile!

To locate a physical therapist who specializes in the pelvic floor:

www.apta.org; Find a therapist, woman's health.

www.pelvicrehab.com Find a pelvic rehabilitation practitioner near you.

Podcasts

For The Mind:

- Sounds True: Insights at the Edge with Tami Simon
- Mind Love with Melissa Monte
- Add Heart with Deborah Rozman, PhD

For the Body:

- The Girl Friend Doctor show with Dr. Anna Cabecca, MD
- Tight-lipped

Medical providers for products and services:

Spectra Wellness Solutions: Dr. Lisa Saff Koche, MD; Behavior Medicine Specialist, Author of Get Lit; Tampa Bay, FL specializing in Integrative and Functional Medicine.

Services and products to address almost all medical and health needs.

Dr. Anna Cabecca, DO, OBGYN, FACOG Sexual CPR, numerous books of interest, products to address a multitude of woman's concerns; Absolutely the best resource for Menopause.

Odela Health Virtual visits for vaginal estrogen and Sex Coaching.

Clear Passage Physical Therapy in Gainsville, Florida for female infertility, bowel conditions, adhesions and internal scar tissue, and chronic pain.

Websites of Interest referenced in the book

Recommended products:

1. www.intimaterose.com For products and informational videos by Dr. Amanda Olsen, DPT, PRPC; Author of Restoring Your Pelvic Floor for Women.
2. www.ohnut.com for Stretchy 4 ring buffer to address pain with deep penetration and the Pelvic gym for educational videos of all things pelvic by pelvic health physical therapist.

For the heart and the mind:

1. www.heartmath.org A wealth of resources to live a heart-centered life.
2. www.soundstruefoundation.org A host of resources for mindfulness, self-compassion, and other wisdom-based teachings.
3. www.rhythmofregulation.com Hosted by Deb Dana, LCSW for mindfulness training and polyvagal guided living.
4. www.wimhoffmethod.com Practical ways to become happier, healthier, and stronger.

Getting to know your vulva, clitoris, and pelvic floor:

1. www.labiallibrary.org.au Real pictures of real women to help you embrace your lady parts.
2. www.sophiawallaceart.com and www.yesclitercy.com Best resources to learn about the Clitoris.
3. www.theflowerempowered.com Numerous resources for dealing with pelvic floor dysfunctions by the author of Empower Your Flower, qualified yoga instructor and personal trainer, Denise Conway.

Tips for the bedroom:

1. www.missjaiya.com Discover your sexual blueprint type and superpower. Take a quick 5 min quiz to unlock the pleasure you're looking or go deeper with the full test and sexual coaching.
2. www.greatsexguidance.com Michael Castleman, Author of Sizzling Sex for Life, Journalist, and sex

counselor; also offers a Great Sex Guidance Weekly Newsletter and blogs 2x month on Psychology Today. com All About Sex.

A non-profit with a heart for pelvic health:

www.tightlipped.org A grassroots movement by and for people with chronic vulvovaginal and pelvic pain.

Note: A portion of the proceeds of this book are being donated to their cause and mission.

Recommended Reading List:

For health and wellness:

1. Get Lit: Simple Answers to Overcome Exhaustion, Escape Stress, Harness Limitless Energy and Ignite Your Inner Athlete by Dr. Lisa Saff Koche, MD, ABAARM.

For a deeper understanding of sexuality and the mind/body connection:

1. Come As You Are: The Surprising New Science That Will Transform Your Sex Life by Emily Nagoski, Ph.D.
2. Sex Points: Reclaim Your Sex Life with the Revolutionary Mult-Point System by Dr. Bat Sheva Marcus Ph.D.
3. Sizzling Sex for Life: Everything You Need to Know to Maximize Erotic Pleasure At Any Age by Micheal Castleman.

For mental health and a better understanding of your central nervous system:

1. The Untethered Soul: A Journey Beyond Yourself by Michael Singer; Check out Temple of the Universe for inspirational weekly talks by Michael.
2. Anchored, How to Befriend Your Nervous System using the Polyvagal System, Deb Dana, LCSW.

Consult with Me

In so far as services offered:

1. Individualized In-Person Evaluations and Treatment Sessions.
2. Video Consults/Coaching.

Conditions we treat:

1. WOMEN'S HEALTH: Pelvic pain, painful intercourse, prenatal/postpartum conditions and education, urinary or fecal incontinence, constipation/slow transit digestion, organ prolapse, post abdominal/mastectomy surgery recovery, bladder conditions like over active or difficulty emptying, low back, SI joint or tailbone/rectal pain.
2. MEN'S HEALTH: Pelvic pain, urinary and fecal incontinence, post prostatectomy recovery, bladder conditions like pain, over active or difficulty emptying, rectal/tailbone pain, constipation/slow transit digestion,

groin pain, post abdominal surgery recovery, low back pain.

3. LGBTQ+: Post gender affirmation surgery recovery and guidance Painful intercourse, rectal pain.

Acknowledgment

Many thanks to the following people in my life. You are all a gift!

Dr. Lisa Koche, MD, friend, and medical colleague, for writing the forward to this book. You are a gift to all those who know you and your light leads many to a path of healing and wholeness.

Gregg Gonzales with The Speak Easy Method. Thanks for helping me get the ball rolling on the book writing journey and holding space for me in the process.

To my friend, **Alicia Durigan** who graciously volunteered to be the photographer for my book. Thanks for capturing all those great images, making us look good, and as always, making us laugh.

To **Caroline Mallon** who allowed me to use her as a model in demonstrating the stretches for the all-important home exercise program. I graciously thank you for joining me in spreading the news about this all-important condition.

To **Larry** and **Belinda Wurn** for leading me down the road less traveled and giving me a safe place to land during a pivotal time in my life.

To **Melissa Shubert**, PT, mentor, and dear friend for always being there to encourage me along the way, offering sage advice and wisdom.

To **Tim McKenna**, my partner, and best friend, that listened to every word in this book multiple times. He knows more about this subject matter than many should. I appreciate your devotion and constant support in all my endeavors. You are a rock!

And finally, to all my patients who trusted me with their stories and their health. Every day you teach me and inspire me!

About the Author

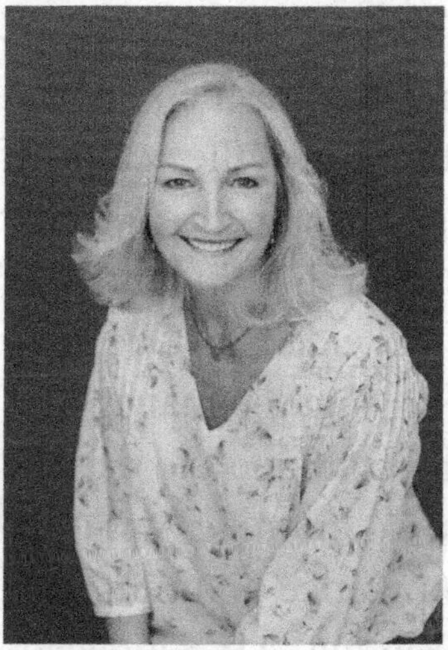

The author recalls her childhood when people asked, "What do you want to be when you grow up?" Her response at that time was a simple desire to help people. Little did she know that this aspiration would lead her to a heartfelt and beautiful career in Physical Therapy.

At the age of sixteen, she knew she wanted to become a physical therapist. Enrolling in a career exploration class during high school, she felt guided to interview professionals in this field, driven by a sense of grace. None of her classmates' presentations resonated with her like her own. From that day forward, she was resolute in her ambition to become a Physical Therapist. However, reaching this goal was a long and challenging journey. After pursuing various paths in cosmology, medical assisting, and personal training, she eventually realized her dream at the age of thirty-four in 1993, when she graduated from the Medical College of Georgia in Augusta. The choices, challenges, and lessons along her journey made her more determined and shaped her into a better person. She now views her profession as a vocation—a true calling she is grateful for daily. Waking up with the question, "What can I do to make someone's life better today?" she sees her childhood dream come to fruition.

Transitioning into a personal perspective, she describes her early career in a hospital setting, where she gained foundational knowledge. However, she found her greatest satisfaction in treating patients at an outpatient facility. These patients primarily had orthopedic diagnoses. Guided by a mentor who specialized in manual therapy, she ventured into the realm of outpatient care, joining a company managed by a well-respected manual therapist. Not only did he support her in pursuing manual therapy, but the company also provided an excellent clinic management training program. Becoming the manager of one of Metro Atlanta's largest clinics, she continued to expand her expertise through education, including training with Dr. Stanley Paris. She then opened her own practice and remained independently employed in Cumming, Georgia. After a decade in business, a significant change was on the horizon.

The story takes a personal turn as she reflects on her twenty-four-year marriage. One day, she looked in the mirror and wondered where she had gone. Like many women, she had lost herself, prioritizing others' needs over her own. She recognized the pattern of sacrificing her voice, true feelings, and personal boundaries to please others. This path of least resistance led to a loss of confidence and identity. After six years of soul-searching, she mustered the strength to leave the marriage. Though difficult, she knew she needed to follow her heart, which led her to a place of renewed strength and self-discovery. She emphasizes the importance of patience during periods of waiting and the courage required to embrace change and venture into the unknown.

Believing that people and circumstances have a purpose, she recalls signing up for a Yoga Teacher Training Certification program in December of 2017. This decision aligned with her journey of self-discovery. The training introduced her to a transformative book recommended by a classmate, "The Untethered Soul: The Journey Beyond Yourself" by Michael Singer. This book provided her with insights into managing thoughts and emotions, finding inner peace, and connecting with her true self. The book also encouraged her to let go and trust life's path. Inspired by the book, she took a chance on an opportunity in Gainesville, Florida, and discovered Clear Passage Physical Therapy, a clinic founded by Larry and Belinda Wurn. The Wurns' unique manual therapy technique, the Wurn Method, deeply resonated with her. Training with them led her to specialize in Women's Health.

The author then explains her motivation for writing a book about painful intercourse. While she had wanted to write a book for years, she hadn't settled on a topic until a moment of inspiration by the beach. Recognizing the lack of comprehensive information on this topic, she felt compelled to address the gap. Her goal is to provide readers with educational insights, practical self-care strategies, and a more open dialogue about painful intercourse. She aims to empower readers, replacing mystery, shame, and embarrassment with knowledge and actionable steps toward a happier life, intimacy, and fulfillment.

Contact the author at:
www.shor.by/sandismith

Made in United States
North Haven, CT
10 November 2026

22091346R00114